# The Fitness Protocols

## Look Better, Feel Better, and Live a Better Life

### Epi Torres

The Fitness Protocols

ISBM 978-0-615-48716-8

I dedicate this book to my mother and father.
Thanks for laying the foundation of my success.

# Preface

This book is a practical guide for people who want help accomplishing lasting weight loss and fitness improvement, and are ready to do it.

This is not a typical weight loss, fitness, or diet book — it is a unique, comprehensive, and easy-to-follow guide designed to help you overcome the common issues that make lasting weight loss and fitness improvement so difficult to accomplish.

The content is primarily based on the lessons I learned, and the knowledge I acquired over the nine years since I lost, and have successfully kept seventy-five pounds off.

I had struggled because of my poor fitness for a while before I lost the weight. I was a typical yo-yo dieter. My weight struggle started about one year or so after I quit smoking in 1984. I remember joining my first diet program when I was living in Connecticut around 1986. Thereafter, I remember entering into what I recall were bi-annual yo-yo cycles. I would typically lose weight during the summer and would regain it all back and then some during the winter. I did that year in and year out.

I reached my tipping point at 250 pounds and a 44-inch waist to boot. It was not pretty. My fitness was very poor. I had low energy, not much strength, poor flexibility, and little to no stamina. My day-to-day life was not very joyful. I had a hard time just doing the basic things like bending down to put my socks on and tying my shoes.

Then one day, fed up with my fitness condition, and disgusted with the image I saw in the mirror, I made a decision to make a change for good. One year and a few months later, I had dropped 70 pounds of body weight and ten inches had come off my waist.

In order to find a long-term solution, I did a lot of homework and sought the help of a number of professionals. I read many books and articles, and I hired a fitness coach, a dietician, and even a psychologist to help me find the best way. In the process, I learned a lot about nutrition and the human body and the mind. Just about a year after I had lost the weight, I started to write a book about it. I have finally completed the book after nine years of experience maintaining the original weight loss. This is a claim that apparently very few can make. I hope what we have put together will help you conquer your struggle with fitness.

I wish you the best of luck!

# Acknowledgments

This book would not be possible if it were not for a bunch of people who contributed.

I appreciate Janet Gualtieri for her long-term support of this book project.

I appreciate Megan Branning, Paul Furiga, Ricardo J. Torres, and Jessica Antoszyk for their efforts researching, writing, and editing the initial book version.

I appreciate Kelsic Pross for her support and advice on this, many other writing, and marketing efforts, we have worked on together.

I appreciate Rob Brown, Chris Foot, and the rest of the team for making things go so well at Remote DBA Experts while I took time to finish the book.

I appreciate Mihaela Enos for her feedback and suggestions on portions of the content.

I appreciate Gail Cato for her editing effort and kind feedback.

I hope I did not forget anyone. If I did, I sincerely apologize!

# Table of Contents

Introduction ......................................................................... 1

Commitment ......................................................................... 7

    Build Your Readiness ........................................................ 10

    Step 1 - Power and Control Capabilities ............................. 12

    Step 2 - Economic Capabilities ......................................... 15

    Step 3 - Health Capabilities ............................................. 20

    Step 4 - Support Capabilities ............................................ 23

    Step 5 - Readiness Assurance ........................................... 26

    Building Your Conviction ................................................. 30

    Step 1 - Drawbacks ......................................................... 33

    Step 2 - Risks ................................................................. 37

    Step 3 - Consequences ..................................................... 53

    Step 4 - Other Not Wanted ............................................... 58

    Step 5 - Possibilities ........................................................ 60

    Step 6 - Impact .............................................................. 68

    Step 7 - Needs ................................................................ 70

    Step 8 - Other Wanted ..................................................... 72

    Step 9 - Conviction Assurance ........................................... 74

    The Formal Commitment ................................................. 80

Preparation .......................................................................... 85

Learn the Basics ........................................................................88

How the Mind Works ...............................................................90

How the Body Works ............................................................. 107

Key Takeaways ........................................................................ 141

Establish Your Baseline ......................................................... 144

Step 1 - Your Current Conditions ....................................... 145

Step 2 - Finding the Root Reasons ...................................... 158

Develop Your Strategy ........................................................... 165

Step 1 - Set Your Key Targets .............................................. 167

Step 2 - Develop Your Strategy ............................................ 171

Step 3 - Device Your Plans ................................................... 175

Plan 1 - Lifestyle Adjustment and Management Plan ......... 177

Plan 2 - Nutritional Adjustment and Management Plan ..... 182

Plan 3 - Physical Activity Adjustment and Management Plan ...... 188

Plan 4 - Setup and Integration Plan .................................... 193

The Setup and Integration Plan ........................................... 196

Change ..................................................................................... 199

Forge ........................................................................................ 227

Observe .................................................................................... 232

Appraise ................................................................................... 237

Tweak ....................................................................................... 241

Maintenance..................................................................................245

Maintenance Strategy.................................................................248

Techniques, Tools, and Tricks...................................................252

# Introduction

Congratulations for your decision to improve your fitness, and your choice of Fitness Protocols™ to help you accomplish your goal! For this purpose, "fitness" is the ideal level of physical condition that enables you to look and feel good while meeting the physical and mental demands required by the tasks in your most important roles in life. Depending on what people must do or like to do, they have different fitness level needs. Athletes have very different fitness level needs than homemakers, people who work in a physically demanding job, or those who work in less physically demanding ones. Our goal is to help you become as fit as necessary to meet your specific wants and needs and make your life more joyful and fulfilling.

You are about to embark on a very interesting and unique journey to improve your life! Whether you have attempted this before or this is your first time, this program should be a unique and rewarding experience for you. Besides the benefits related to the specific area of fitness, the exercises you are about to complete can benefit you a multitude of ways. The program we have designed is unique. It takes advantage of a number of proven successful approaches in several areas. This is not necessarily new material we have invented or made up. We base our approach on proven theories and science, and have integrated it to enable the process required to accomplish lasting change. The goal is to make it much easier to accomplish your fitness improvement goal. We hope you will find it effective and ultimately fruitful. Keep in mind that change is a journey and not a destination per se. We hope to make the journey more pleasant and less bumpy than it would have otherwise been without our guidance.

## You Are Not Alone

If you are like most of us who struggle with fitness issues, you may have already attempted to get in better shape in the past. This is normal and you should not feel too bad about it! In fact, you are not alone. According to several studies, over 90% of those who attempt to get and stay in better shape fail to do so. Of the small percent that are successful at it, the majority had attempted to get in shape and failed five to seven times before they were ultimately successful. However, please do not despair; we intend to change that with this approach. If you follow along, it should take a lot less effort than these studies have shown.

### What Got Us Here

Many factors have influenced the reasons why so many of us are out of shape these days. However, the bottom line is that we consume excess calories and we do not burn enough of them. Moreover, no matter what anyone says, it is all about the calories. Calories are the units of measure of the energy humans need to survive. Each of our bodies requires so many calories to survive every day. We obtain them from the food and drinks we consume and we burn them when our bodies are in motion. When we take in more calories than those we burn, the extra calories are stored as fat; if we consume enough of them we gain weight at whatever rate we do that. Similarly, when we burn more calories than we take in, we can lose weight. It is that simple!

### Less Activity

A number of factors have led many of us to become more sedentary. Much more of what we do to earn a living requires less physical activity. We use cars and other transportation means to go everywhere. We do much more shopping on TV and the Web. We watch TV, play video games, do social media, and surf the Web instead of moving outdoors.

### And More Food

On top of being less active, we are eating more. The cost of food has decreased and its availability has dramatically increased. Fast and relatively cheap food is available everywhere and almost anytime. It has become so convenient and inexpensive that many people dine out more than they cook meals at home. Time constraints and convenience also drive fast-food consumption both from the typical outlets and from new sources at the regular grocery store. Eating out typically means higher caloric consumption further adding insult to injury.

Introduction

Ending the Fitness Struggle

Why is it such a struggle? Why does change seem so hard to achieve? Let us begin by examining some of the key factors that contribute to the problem, starting our struggle with fitness. First, most people do not truly understand the powerful impact and multiple benefits of fitness. Therefore, they may not feel as motivated to pursue fitness improvement with the fervor, priority, and energy it requires and deserves. As in most situations, when we attempt to go after something without a wholehearted effort we fail. Success requires commitment based on understanding the connection between the benefits of improved fitness and a much higher quality of life-better health, relationships, and wealth.

Second, the current approaches to fitness improvement are fragmented, and they lack a comprehensive approach. Most of these approaches (plans, programs, etc.) take a very narrow view of the problem and the challenges faced by those struggling with fitness. Companies offering "solutions" to our fitness struggle seem to just want to sell us books, memberships, food, medications, treatments, surgery, and/or some type of equipment. It is a multibillion-dollar annual market and with no end in sight. Many of them have one mission: to take your money and run. Moreover, they usually leave you right where you started, and sometimes-even worse-out of shape and struggling all over again.

Let us examine a typical approach to getting in shape. Many motives drive us to attempt to get in better shape. So whatever the motive is we tend to jump right into some kind of action after we decide to do something about it. We usually get into some diet (of the month) and/or start doing some form of exercise. Some of us may seek professional help and others just ask friends or family members what worked for them. Some may buy books or seek information on the Web to help them along the way. So what happens? We may or may not lose weight because of our effort. If we lose it, we may or may not keep it off for the long term. We tend to bounce back to our old habits and routines over some time and slowly but surely, we gain weight-sometimes more weight than that we lost. We are unable to sustain the strange diets we get into and the exercise routines that we start. The equipment we purchase ends up becoming a storage apparatus in one of the rooms in the house. In addition, some of the special food we bought for the diet becomes a lab experiment in the fridge or kitchen pantry. Then many of us tend to repeat these cycles. The struggle continues and we often get bigger and out of shape.

Ultimately, in order to end our struggle successfully, we need to adjust the way we live our life. Simplistically speaking, we just have to develop a better approach to enable us to eat better and be more active. The challenge we face is that over time we have developed a set of habits and routines by which we live our life. These are so ingrained in us we are oblivious to them. Thus, we rarely examine them because we are not conscious of them. It is a human version of an autopilot. What we do, when we do it, where we do it, etc. tends to have some routine and/or habit associated with it.

In order to develop a successful better approach we need to examine these routines and habits we live by and we need to evaluate their impact on us and on those we care most about. Once we understand that, we need to determine which we need to adjust, which we need to eliminate, and what new ones we need to create to better serve our new approach.

The Science of Change

Change is a challenging process for humans. According to research conducted over the last few decades by Dr. James O. Prochaska (of the University of Rhode Island) and his colleagues, lasting change requires you to go through several sequential stages:

- Precontemplation stage. At this stage, you are not really thinking about change, do not believe you need to change, or are simply not ready to start changing anytime soon.
- Contemplation stage. At this stage, you want to change, but do not intend to start just yet. Perhaps you want to learn more first, or else you may just do not want it badly enough yet.

- Preparation stage. At this stage, you are ready to start. You are preparing, learning, planning, and maybe even doing a few things.
- Action stage. At this stage, you are actively trying to implement the changes.
- Maintenance stage. At this stage, you have successfully changed, and you are now trying to keep the changes. In this stage, you will actively work to resist relapsing to a prior stage.
- Termination stage. At this stage, change is completed. Habits are formed and set. You will no longer have to work as hard, if at all, to resist relapsing.

Additionally, the research shows it typically takes individuals several attempts to reach the final and successful Termination stage. Confirming this finding, research done by the National Weight Control Registry since 1994, indicates individuals who accomplish lasting fitness improvement relapsed between five and seven times before doing so.

The Right Step at the Right Time

Getting and staying in shape can be much easier to accomplish if you want it badly enough and if you do the right things at the right time. Lacking an approach like the one we offer, only a small percent are able to accomplish sustainable fitness. According to the National Weight Control Registry Study, fewer than 10 percent of those who become fit are able to sustain their new fitness level. Our approach will change that. If you follow along with diligence, you will be able to become and remain fit for good! The process takes time and requires a good dose of patience and perseverance. There are no quick fixes. There are no ways around it. If you really want to become and remain fit, you must go through these stages one-step at a time. If you are successful, the benefits can be plenty!

Our ultimate goal is to ensure you become and remain fit for good in the shortest amount of time possible. We designed Fitness Protocols™ to help you navigate through these seemingly complex stages of change more easily and successfully. More importantly, it will help you minimize the possibility of potential setbacks or total failure.

The Fitness Protocols Process

The following diagram illustrates the process we will guide you through in order to accomplish your goal.

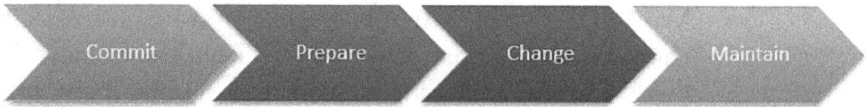

| Commit | Prepare | Change | Maintain |
|--------|---------|--------|----------|

We designed our approach around four key protocols to help you accomplish this. The Commitment Protocol is the first and most critical step in the process. It will help you ensure your decision to improve your fitness is solid and highly sustainable. Your commitment and determination are critical to your success. The adage "Where there is a will there is an A" is highly applicable here. The stronger your conviction, the higher the probability you will reach your goal and the easier it will seem to get it accomplished. Once you feel you have reached a strong sense of commitment, you will move on to the Preparation Protocol. Here we help you get ready to accomplish the necessary changes in your approach to fitness. When you feel you have mustered enough commitment and are ready to move forward, you will move on to the Change Protocol. Here we will help you implement a new approach to help you succeed. Finally, you will move on to the fourth and final Maintenance Protocol. Here we help you ensure the new approach sticks and forms into habits. Once it takes hold, the chances of relapse become less and less over time, making it much easier to remain fit for good!

We have designed a flexible approach so that any point in the process you may go back one or more stages to get reinforcement if necessary. We have broken down the book's main sections accordingly. Each section consists of information and exercises intended to help you accomplish the main purpose of the corresponding approach step.

# Commitment

This protocol will help you develop highly sustainable commitment to improve and maintain your fitness for the rest of your life.

About Commitment

Commitment is a critical success factor in this process because it is what ultimately powers and sustains your determination. Determination is ultimately, what will to see you though the four key stages of the Fitness Protocols™ process shown in the figure below.

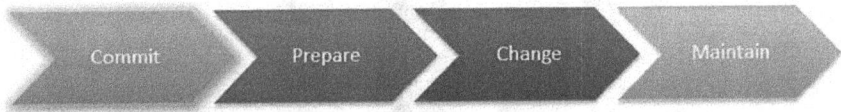

Building Sustainable Commitment

Since you are reading this, you have obviously developed a certain level of motivation for better fitness. The question is whether it is adequate to see you through to the end of the process or not. Will you be able to improve and then sustain the improvement made? As you read in our main introduction, doing so is something very few are able to. That is the reason why building sustainable commitment is so critical for anyone attempting effortful goals!

The Dynamics of Commitment

Building commitment involves managing the dynamic tension between two key forces:

- Drivers
- Pushbacks

Drivers are the forces that compel you toward commitment and pushbacks are those that deter you from it. This type of dynamic tension is often active in most decision-making processes. The bigger the decision is, the more complex its structure and the stronger the tension that builds between these forces. The diagram below illustrates how this dynamic works in this context.

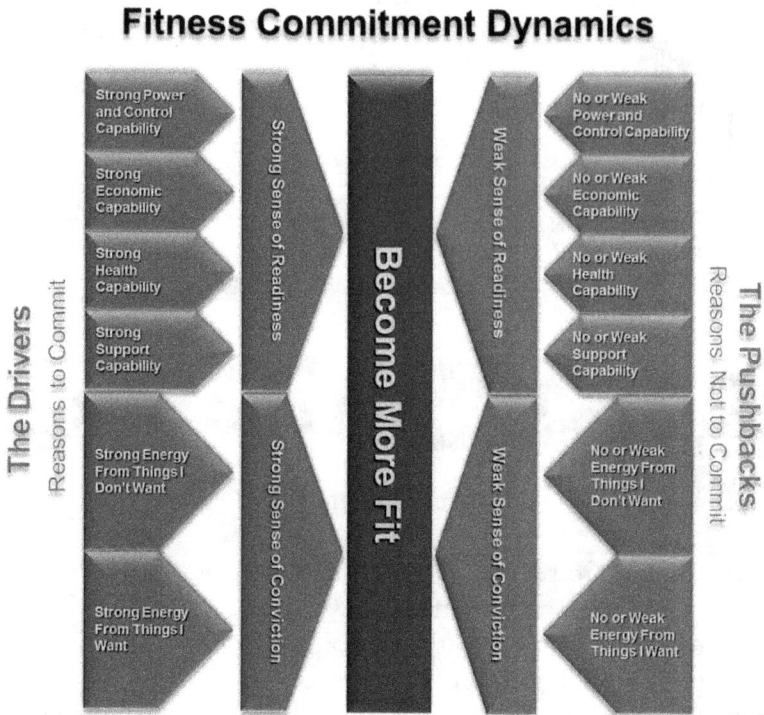

## Fitness Commitment Dynamics

| The Drivers — Reasons to Commit | | | | The Pushbacks — Reasons Not to Commit | | |
|---|---|---|---|---|---|---|
| Strong Power and Control Capability | Strong Sense of Readiness | Become More Fit | Weak Sense of Readiness | No or Weak Power and Control Capability | | |
| Strong Economic Capability | | | | No or Weak Economic Capability | | |
| Strong Health Capability | | | | No or Weak Health Capability | | |
| Strong Support Capability | | | | No or Weak Support Capability | | |
| Strong Energy From Things I Don't Want | Strong Sense of Conviction | | Weak Sense of Conviction | No or Weak Energy From Things I Don't Want | | |
| Strong Energy From Things I Want | | | | No or Weak Energy From Things I Want | | |

Driving forces on the left-hand side of the diagram include those factors that drive your sense of readiness and conviction and any other factors not included in the first two.

Pushback forces on the right-hand side of the diagram include those factors that drive a weak sense of readiness and or conviction, and any other factors not included in the first two.

To build highly sustainable commitment, you will first need to eliminate or mitigate as many pushbacks as you possibly can. Once you feel ready, you will identify the most meaningful set of highly energizing drivers possible.

# Commitment

## The Power of Emotional Energy

Our goal here is to harness as much energy as possible. We will need lots of the negative energy produced by the drawbacks, risks, negative consequences, and any other things you do not want from being out of shape. In addition, we need lots of the positive energy produced by the excitement from imagining all the possibilities, the positive impact of the needs you can meet with improved fitness, and from any other things, you want from your improved fitness condition. To help harness the most energy, we will help you explore the most meaningful reasons to accomplish and sustain fitness improvement whether they relate to feeling or looking better, getting more things done, or other meaningful goals. Once harnessed, the energy will propel you and help you progress and overcome obstacles.

In the end, success requires that you find the best positive and negative reasons to improve your fitness. Regardless of their polarity, they must be highly meaningful to you. You must really dislike the negatives and really want the positive ones. While this is about you and no one else, others may provide impetus for action. For example, your love for someone and the strong desire to be there for him or her may provide the strongest reason, thus becoming one of your best sources of energy to take action, persist, persevere, and sustain the gains made.

We are looking for goose bumps to come out of here. You need to feel highly compelled to do this! You need HIGH levels of sustainable energy day in and day out. Without it, you will become another statistic. One of millions who set goals and never get them done or who reach the goal but then lose impetus and end up back or even worse off than where they started. If you do not get the energy, do not waste your time and effort. Keep looking for it until you find it. Then nothing will stop you! NOTHING!

## Build Your Readiness

This part will help you build a strong sense of readiness to pursue and accomplish your goal.

About Readiness

Your sense of readiness is the powerful feeling that you are ready to take this task on. This is the first part because it makes no sense to move forward if you are not quite ready. You must feel a strong sense that you can do this or it will not happen, thus wasting your time and money and getting disappointed, perhaps one more time, that you did not accomplish your goal.

In the following section, we will help you evaluate and if necessary build your sense of readiness. Once you feel it is feasible and you are ready to do it, you can then move on to the next part of the protocol where you will build a strong sense of conviction.

The Key Aspects of Readiness

Readiness for this effort depends on four key aspects:

- Power and control aspects
- Economic aspects
- Health aspects
- Support aspects

Power and control aspects involve your capability to make and sustain key decisions for the effort. Economic aspects involve your capability to afford and pay your best attention to the overall effort. Health aspect involves your capability to perform physical activities and make adjustments to what and how you eat. Finally, support aspects refer to your capability to get and retain the support of key individuals and to set up and maintain supportive environments. We will delve into the details in each section that follows. The figure below shows how these four aspects align to drive a strong sense of readiness in you.

Strong Power and Control Capability

Strong Economic Capability

Strong Health Capability

Strong Support Capability

Strong Sense of Readiness

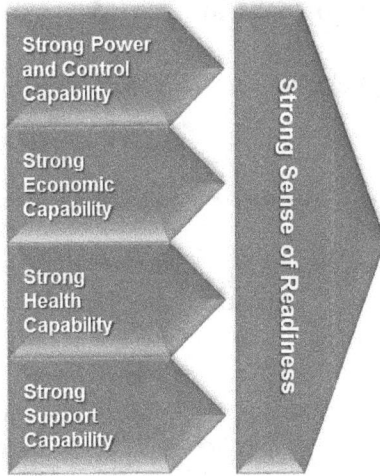

As mentioned before, this is a critical aspect! Your sense of readiness is very important and should be carefully evaluated and developed before moving on to the next section.

Before moving on, let us make one important clarification about your sense of readiness. Typically, there is never a "perfect time" to do things. In this case, we will not be exploring for simple or usual issues that could provide excuses for never moving forward. Here, we are mostly interested in a few real "showstoppers"-the type that could impede sustainable change, regardless of your level of conviction for the goal.

To ensure your success, we do not recommend proceeding any further until you feel truly ready after completing the following five steps.

**NOTE: If it is clear that none of these are an issue for you, you may skip this section and go right to building you conviction on page 24.**

## Step 1 - Power and Control Capabilities

This step will help you evaluate your current power and control capabilities.

Assessing Power and Control Capability

Your sense of power and ability to control certain aspects of this effort are key ingredients to success. For our purpose, power means a sense of the ability or capability to make meaningful decisions or act on them. Feeling powerless means lacking, at least in your mind, the authority, or capacity to decide or act on a decision. People who feel powerless in situations tend to use the following terms to describe the feeling: hamstrung, handcuffed, helpless, high and dry, paralyzed, weak, and impotent. When you feel others can override or strongly influence you one-way or the other at any time, it means your power capability should be considered low for the particular item being considered. Parents, superiors, siblings, partners, children, spouses, etc. can exert power over us directly or indirectly, thus making us less able to perform important process tasks effectively.

On the other hand, control means a sense of authority or high influence over someone or something. Feeling in control means we feel in charge and capable of making any determinations regarding what we are in control of. In life, there are many aspects that are within our control and many outside of it. Moreover, most, if not all, of those things within our control have to do with us.

Getting Ready

The following questions should help you think and prepare before completing the exercise below. When doing this, try to rely on the most recent past experiences possible. Try to recall how you have typically tended to deal with similar or identical situations. There is no right or wrong answer here-this is just for your consumption. The more honest you are the better for you. Remember, this is a critical aspect!

- Have you been able to make and sustain effortful decisions in the past?
- Is there anyone else who needs to be involved in this decision-making process?
- Can you make the decision and sustain it on your own?
- Have you been able to change any habits successfully before?
- Have you been able to say NO to self or to others?
- Have you been able to move away and stay away from temptations and distractions?
- How much control have you had over your time?
- How much "free" time have you had lately?
- How much time can you easily allocate to focus on this effort?
- Have you been able to set routines and keep a consistent schedule for prolonged periods?

Power and Control Assessment

Use the form on the following page to assess your power and control capability. Use your gut feeling to rate your capability on a 1-5 scale. A "1" means you feel you have no capability and a "5" means you feel fully capable. Later on in the book, we will ask you to consider developing a strategy to help you increase your capability on items you rate below a "3."

If you prefer a larger copy, you may download it from www.fitnessprotocols.com/book/forms.pdf.

| Key Power and Control Aspects | Ability Level | | | | |
|---|---|---|---|---|---|
| | 1 | 2 | 3 | 4 | 5 |
| Ability and power to make and sustain decisions | 1 | 2 | 3 | 4 | 5 |
| Ability and power to change and maintain eating habits | 1 | 2 | 3 | 4 | 5 |
| Ability and power to say "no" to distractions or temptations | 1 | 2 | 3 | 4 | 5 |
| Ability and power to change and maintain exercise habits | 1 | 2 | 3 | 4 | 5 |
| Ability and power to allocate the required time to the efforts | 1 | 2 | 3 | 4 | 5 |
| Ability and power to change and manage your environments | 1 | 2 | 3 | 4 | 5 |
| Ability and power to pay attention and focus on the efforts | 1 | 2 | 3 | 4 | 5 |
| Ability and power to set and follow a consistent schedule | 1 | 2 | 3 | 4 | 5 |

## Step 2 - Economic Capabilities

This step should help you evaluate your economic capabilities.

Determining Your Economic Capability

Having economic capability means possessing available funds and then the ability and power to spend them on several expenses this effort will require. Also and very important, it is being free from stress produced by personal and business financial issues. The effort to get in better shape will require money for food, new clothing, equipment, etc. The amount will vary depending on your situation, personality, and level of creativity. For example, a person who needs/wants to reduce thirty pounds will spend less than one who needs/wants to lose seventy. On the other hand, a person who likes good things will spend on fancy exercise clothing while others are fine with the shorts they already have. A creative person will make weight out of water bottles while others may buy new dumbbells from a store. A key success factor in this program will be to give away clothing after it does not fit and to purchase the next size down just before you have arrived at it. These things will take some funds and if you do not have them, it will create challenges that may set you back.

Getting Ready

Getting in shape will require investment. The level of investment required will depend on your situation, level of taste and affordability, level of creativity and resourcefulness, and the quantity and quality of the items and services you decide to invest in. According to your specific situation, you need to consider investing in:

- Professional advice and support: doctors, personal coaches, trainers, or other professionals.
- Memberships in fitness clubs, classes, Web-based programs, etc.
- Clothing and fitness apparel.
- Food, food preparation items, and supplements.
- Fitness equipment and gear.
- Learning materials and references.

The above comprehensive list will give you an idea of what things you need to consider.

The form on the following page provides a place for you to estimate the level of investment you feel you will need to make to support this important effort.

Keep in mind as you do this that there are also a number of potential short-term and long-term savings you need to consider before you establish the net economic effect, and perhaps the return on investment for those more financially avid. This does not have to be super accurate.

If you prefer a larger copy, you may download it from www.fitnessprotocols.com/book/forms.pdf.

# Commitment

| Item | Quantity | Amount/Month | Total |
|---|---|---|---|
| Professional advice and support | | | |
| Memberships | | | |
| Clothing and fitness apparel | | | |
| Food, food preparation items, and supplements | | | |
| Fitness equipment and gear | | | |
| Learning material and references | | | |

Having this information will provide a factual basis to help make the following assessment more accurate.

Economic Assessment

Use the form on the following page to assess your economic capabilities. Use your gut feeling to rate your capability on a 1-5 scale. A "1" means you feel you have no capability and a "5" means you feel fully capable. Later on in the book, we will ask you to consider developing a strategy to help you increase your capability on items you rate below a "3."

If you prefer a larger copy, you may download it from www.fitnessprotocols.com/book/forms.pdf.

| Key Economic Aspects | Ability Level | | | | |
|---|---|---|---|---|---|
| | 1 | 2 | 3 | 4 | 5 |
| Availability of sufficient money needed to fund effort | 1 | 2 | 3 | 4 | 5 |
| Freedom from personal or business stress-bearing economic concerns | 1 | 2 | 3 | 4 | 5 |
| Ability and power to allocate and spend available funds | 1 | 2 | 3 | 4 | 5 |

## Step 3 - Health Capabilities

This step will help you evaluate your health capabilities.

Determining Your Health Capabilities

Having health capability means that you have the minimal mental and physical ability necessary to undertake the required effort. Limited ability to undertake these efforts will further challenge you and increase the chances of a setback.

Certain medical conditions, illnesses, and injuries can prevent or limit your effective effort. It is important that you are cognizant of that. Sometimes we are not even aware we may have a certain condition. That is why, if you have not done so yet, getting a baseline full medical exam done before undertaking this effort would be very beneficial and is highly recommended.

**NOTE: Please do not delve into this or any other fitness-related effort before being cleared by your doctor. Make sure she or he agrees you are fit enough to do so.**

Getting Ready

The following definitions may help to understand better the aspects on the assessment form.

Physical strength efforts involve any effort aimed at enhancing your muscular system. Some level of muscular exercises will be required to enhance your fitness. Muscles are important because they are the key to enhancing our ability to burn calories. The reason is that muscles are much more efficient at burning calories than fat. Building them will proportionally increase your metabolism, thus enhancing your ability to lose weight and keep it off. Please note that this does not mean that you need to become a body builder in order to obtain a benefit. Moreover, as you will learn in a later section, becoming stronger is one of the key benefits of fitness improvement. Moreover, gaining physical strength has a number of additional benefits we will explore later.

Cardiovascular fitness involves efforts aimed at enhancing the cardiovascular system, which includes the heart, lungs, and blood vessels. An enhanced system enables a more efficient supply of oxygenated blood to working muscles and the ability of muscles to use the oxygen delivered by the blood supply as a source of energy for movement. If you go up a couple of flights of stairs and you end up huffing and puffing, your cardiovascular capacity is most likely what it should be. Measuring the time it takes you to recover after doing any heavy muscle-using activity is another way to measure how fit you are.

Physical flexibility fitness efforts involve any effort aimed at enhancing muscular flexibility. Muscular flexibility gives us the ability to do even mundane day-to-day tasks with much more ease and less pain. Yoga practices provide a great example of moves aimed at making you highly flexible. There is no need to become a Yogi in order to gain more flexibility and benefit greatly from being highly flexible.

Health Assessment

Use the form on the following page to assess your health capabilities. Use your gut feeling to rate your capability on a 1-5 scale. A "1" means you feel you have no capability and a "5" means you feeling fully capable. Later on in the book, we will ask you to consider developing a strategy to help you increase your capability on items you rate below a "3."

If you prefer a larger copy, you may download it from www.fitnessprotocols.com/book/forms.pdf.

| Key Health Aspects | Ability Level | | | | |
|---|---|---|---|---|---|
| Ability to undertake physical strength fitness efforts | 1 | 2 | 3 | 4 | 5 |
| Ability to undertake physical cardiovascular efforts | 1 | 2 | 3 | 4 | 5 |
| Ability to undertake physical flexibility efforts | 1 | 2 | 3 | 4 | 5 |

## Step 4 - Support Capabilities

This step will help you evaluate your support capabilities.

Determining Your Support Capabilities

Having support capabilities means having a support system, which includes both relationships and environments. The effort to improve your fitness will most likely involve others, including family and friends. Their support is important to your success. Their lack of support can be detrimental to your effort. When people around you do not support end encourage you in this effort, it will make it significantly more challenging for you. They need to be an integral part of it directly and indirectly, especially early on. In addition to supportive people, a good support system includes environments where you live and work. These are also important! When you operate and live in non-supportive ones, it can make things much harder for you. Supportive environments are ones free from temptations and stress-inducing conditions. They are also set up to support your effort. The food available is the right food for you. The facilities are comfortable and conducive to relaxation and ideally fitness activities that support your fitness effort. Environments are highly critical to success, more so than even supportive people, though sometimes they are one in the same.

Getting Ready

The following definitions may help you better understand the aspects on the assessment form.

Supportive family and friends are those who encourage and support you in your effort. These folks understand your need to do what you want to do and are there to offer help when you ask. They give you the mental and physical space you need; they are highly accommodating, even involving themselves in the process by becoming walking friends and helping you with nutrition and exercise efforts. They are also cheerleaders and celebrators of your success along the way.

A supportive environment is one where tempting food and drinks have been eliminated, at least while new habits are formed. It is one where the right foods and drinks are available at the right time. It is one where preparing and storing food is possible. Where exercise equipment and/or space to improvise are available in case the weather is not conducive to outdoor activity.

Support Assessment

Use the form on the following page to assess your support capabilities. Use your gut feeling to rate your capability on a 1-5 scale. A "1" means you feel you have no capability and a "5" means you feel fully capable. Later on in the book, we will ask you to consider developing a strategy to help you increase your capability on items you rate below a "3."

If you prefer a larger copy, you may download it from www.fitnessprotocols.com/book/forms.pdf.

Commitment

| Key Support Aspects | Ability Level | | | | |
|---|---|---|---|---|---|
| Supportive family | 1 | 2 | 3 | 4 | 5 |
| Supportive friends | 1 | 2 | 3 | 4 | 5 |
| Supportive home environment | 1 | 2 | 3 | 4 | 5 |
| Supportive work environment | 1 | 2 | 3 | 4 | 5 |

## Step 5 - Readiness Assurance

This step will help you ensure you are ready to undertake a fitness improvement effort.

At this point, you will make the final determination to move on to the next section or pursue actions that will make you more ready than you are at this point.

**NOTE: Please keep in mind that it would make no sense to get on with the rest of the program if you are not ready yet.**

Assessment Results

The following portion will guide you through the process of identifying specific aspects to enhance your power and control capabilities where needed.

Ultimately, you need to feel ready regardless of the actual scores. It is imperative that you feel it! Nonetheless, it is usual to feel some trepidation or doubt. It is probably impossible to have 100 percent of the bases covered. So feeling some doubt is OK. If you do not feel quite ready, revisit the section and strategies to improve your situation in those areas where the score is below "3."

Just make sure there are no big red flags or showstoppers for you. You need all the capabilities you can muster to ensure nothing can derail your effort once you get going. You should start only when you feel ready instead of starting when you feel any form of ambivalence due to one or more weak readiness capabilities. If there is anything else that can potentially affect the feasibility of this effort, this is the time to deal with it. If you did not rate any item below a "3" in the prior section, you may skip the next section and turn to the "Build Your Conviction" section on page 24. Otherwise, read on.

Enhancing Your Readiness

Take a moment to go back a look at the items you rated below a "3." Consider each of the low-rated items one by one and spend time thinking of ways in which you can improve your capability for each of them.

You do not need to complete this in one sitting. Take your time to think and, if helpful, involve others to determine each strategy.

Use the form on the following page to help you formulate your strategy. The form is simple. Just write the result you wish to accomplish in the first box. Then think of up to three things you could do to accomplish that.

Repeat the step for each of the items you identified working your way leftward until you get down to specific actions that will make it happen.

If you prefer a larger copy, you may download it from www.fitnessprotocols.com/book/forms.pdf.

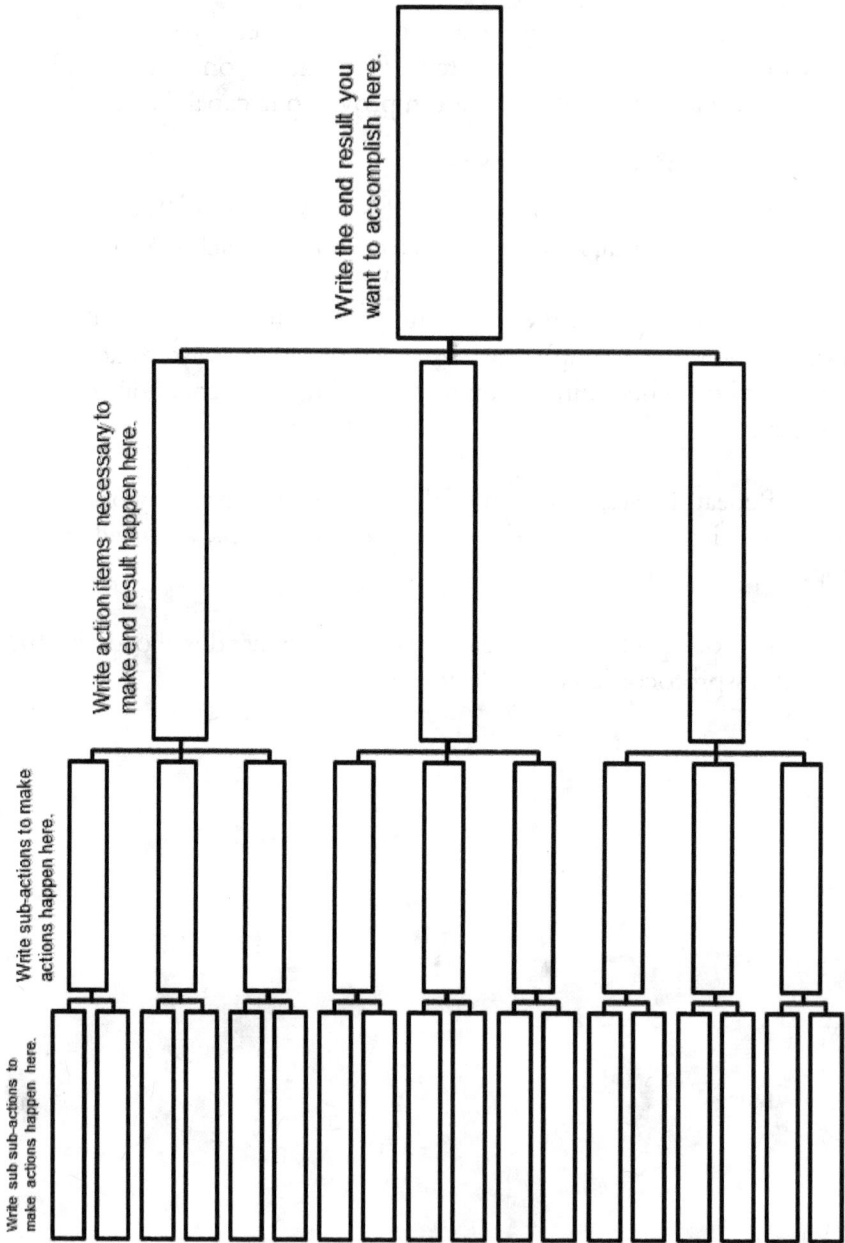

Write the end result you want to accomplish here.

Write action items necessary to make end result happen here.

Write sub-actions to make actions happen here.

Write sub sub-actions to make actions happen here.

Commitment

Once you complete this exercise and you feel you have a handle on all your capabilities you can move on to the next section for building your conviction.

Please keep in mind that while this process takes time to complete, it is crucial. Hang in there for a little longer. This could make the difference between success and failure!

Next, we will move into building your conviction.

## Building Your Conviction

This part will help you build sustainable conviction for fitness improvement and maintenance.

About Conviction

Your sense of conviction is a strong feeling resulting from being highly convinced that you REALLY want to accomplish this task. Conviction results from the process of evaluating and building a strong rationale. To be most successful and to reduce or eliminate any chances of relapsing from one stage to another, or of even failing to accomplish your goal, you should ensure you build the strongest case possible for better fitness.

The Key Aspects of Conviction

Conviction depends on two key aspects:

- Things you don't want
- Things you want

The first key aspect of conviction includes current and future negative aspects associated with your current fitness condition such as:

- Poor fitness drawbacks
- Poor fitness risks
- Poor fitness impact
- Other things you don't want

These are all the things you want get rid of, or avoid. The things you REALLY DISLIKE or hate about being out of shape and would do almost anything to get away from!

The second aspect of conviction includes the positive aspects of improved fitness such as:

- The possibilities of better fitness
- The benefits of better fitness
- The needs better fitness meets
- Other things you want

These are all the positive things you want to obtain by improving your fitness. The things you want REALLY BAD and would do almost anything to get.

The figure below shows how all these forces combine and align to drive your sense of conviction.

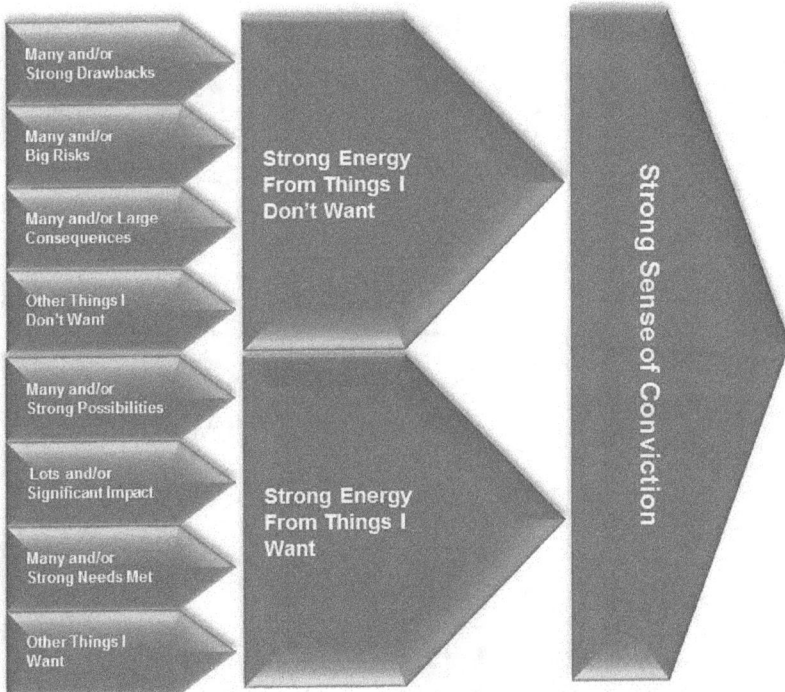

As you can see, emotional energy produced by the things you hate most about being out of shape adds to the energy produced by the things you want most about being in better shape. The resulting energy powers your conviction. This is another important section. Please take your time and make sure you are able to make a strong connection. If you do, nothing will get in your way. This energy will powerfully see you through to the end!

## Step 1 - Drawbacks

Step 1 - Drawbacks

This step will help you identify the worst drawbacks of being out of shape.

About Drawbacks

Drawbacks are objectionable aspects also known as downsides, disadvantages, minuses, or negatives. Identifying and emphasizing these negative aspects can provide significant positive energy for change. For a number of reasons, drawbacks are not always obvious to us. A number of factors affect our level of awareness of drawbacks and our ability to associate them with key aspects of our life's quality. The quality of our life depends on three key factors:

- Our (mental and physical) health
- Our relationship with ourselves and others
- Our emotional and financial wealth

Our fitness level has a significant effect on some or all of these factors. The closer your fitness level is to the one you need to meet the needs of your roles in life, the better the quality of life you should be able to live. Thus, the further away you are the worse it probably is.

The first factor affecting your awareness is the difference (gap) between your current level and the ideal/desired/needed one. The bigger the difference, the more likely you will be able to realize some or all the drawbacks affecting you. The second factor is time. The longer you have been living out of shape, the more used to it you may be and the harder it may be to realize drawbacks. You have "accepted" and gotten used to living with these abnormal conditions; thus, they may not have a motivational effect. However, the fact that you invested in this book says that something got your attention. That is a great start!

## Looking for Your Energy

In this section, we want to elicit as much emotional energy as possible from you. That energy will help ensure your decision to pursue this effort becomes highly sustainable. The following exercise is the first intended to help accomplish that goal. We want to help you realize how your current fitness level is affecting the quality of your life. We will do so by helping you figure out the worst drawbacks related to each key quality of life aspects mentioned above. Once you have a few per each, you will choose the top ones, the ones that seem most important to you. The ones that, if eliminated, will have the biggest effect on your life and the lives of those you care most about. Please take all the time you need for this. This is an important step, as we have said before. You need get the most energy out of it you can. You need to feel very strong emotions when you look at the top items on the resulting list! We are looking for some good old-fashioned goose bumps here! You need to feel strongly about not wanting the drawbacks in your life anymore. Moreover, you need to feel a strong sense that your life would much better without them!

## Loss Avoidance

The reason we have chosen to start with drawbacks is because studies have shown humans tend to obtain a lot more motivation from avoidance of loss than from the possibility of gain.

In the following exercise, you will discover how some of these drawbacks affect your feelings, health, relationships, and wealth.

## Drawbacks Assessment

Complete the form on the following page by answering the questions within it. Once done completing your responses, choose the five worst drawbacks from the list. Simply enter the number 1, 2, 3, 4, or 5 respectively. Use the number "5" to identify the worst drawback and "1" for least of the worst.

If you prefer a larger copy, you may download it from www.fitnessprotocols.com/book/forms.pdf.

| Quality of Life Aspects | | Drawbacks | Rank |
|---|---|---|---|
| How is your fitness affecting you? (your feelings) | 1 | | |
| | 2 | | |
| | 3 | | |
| | 4 | | |
| | 5 | | |
| How is your fitness affecting your health? | 1 | | |
| | 2 | | |
| | 3 | | |
| | 4 | | |
| | 5 | | |
| How is your fitness affecting your relationships? | 1 | | |
| | 2 | | |
| | 3 | | |
| | 4 | | |
| | 5 | | |
| How is your fitness affecting your wealth? | 1 | | |
| | 2 | | |
| | 3 | | |
| | 4 | | |
| | 5 | | |

Think about the worst drawbacks in the context of the people and things you cherish most, and the ways in which fitness can affect them. The success of this exercise depends on your ability to identify the vital few drawbacks that cause you the biggest amount of aggravation. Your success in ranking means you need to feel a strong sense you DO NOT want these drawbacks in your life anymore! Imagine you have a baby in your arms and someone is coming your way with a knife to try to hurt the baby and you. Would you want that? How does that make you feel?-For real, just imagine it happening. That is the type of rejection feelings we want you to feel here. You need to hate these drawbacks-really hate them badly! They are not good for you and those you love and you need to eliminate them!

## Step 2 - Risks

This step will help you identify the most critical risks you run by being out of shape.

About Risks

In the last section, we covered drawbacks or the things we dislike about our situation. In this section, we are going to cover the risk or chance of something bad happening because of poor fitness.

Life is full of risks! Thus, anything can happen to us at any time. The smartest and most successful people think about and work diligently to manage their risks. In this section, we want you to start considering all your fitness-related risks.

Risks are all about the probability and the severity of the outcome as illustrated by the diagram on the following page.

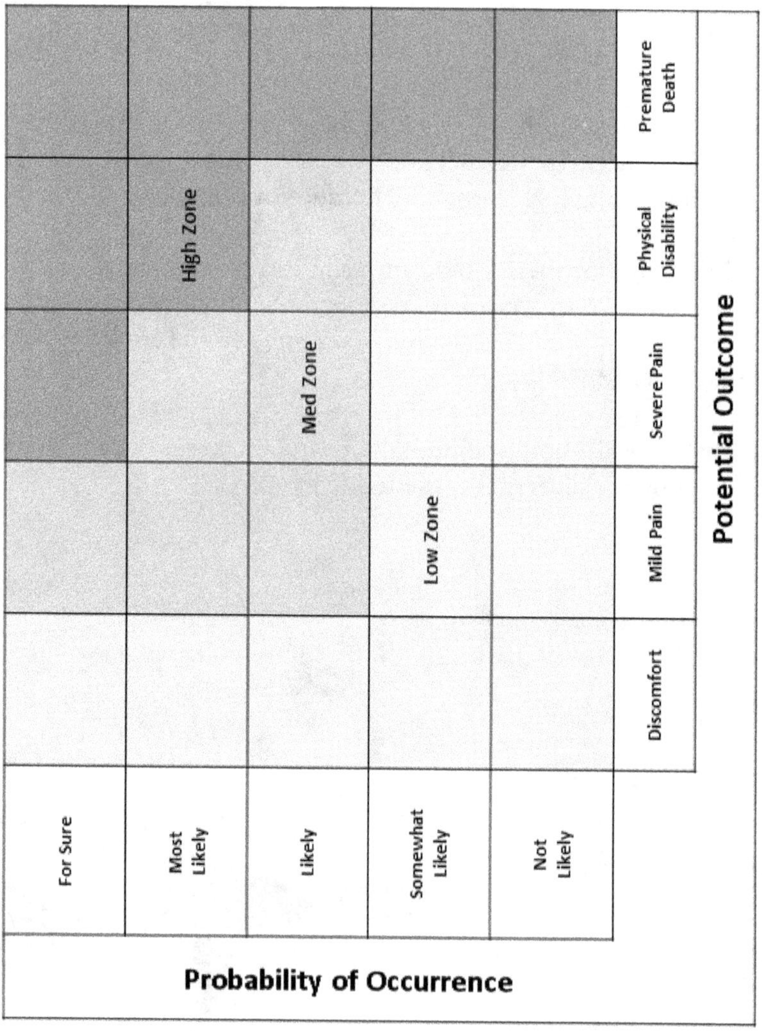
High Zone
Med Zone
Low Zone
Probability of Occurrence
For Sure
Most Likely
Likely
Somewhat Likely
Not Likely
Potential Outcome
Discomfort
Mild Pain
Severe Pain
Physical Disability
Premature Death

The key question asked on any risk assessment is what are the chances of something happening at some point in time and what will happen (worst case) if that happens?

The Risks we want you to consider are categorized according to three key Quality of Life Aspects:

- Your Health
- Your Relationship
- Your Wealth

The idea is to have you consider your poor fitness risks along these three areas. We want you to explore what the risks you are running assuming a poor fitness situation. You will look into what will happen to your health, relationships, and wealth if your fitness is poor or it deteriorates.

Health risks vary according to many factors such as genes or exposure to hazards, and they increase according to your fitness level. The worse your fitness level and the longer you have been out of shape, the higher the risks.

Health risks include:

- Illness
- Injury
- Death

Many things come to play when it comes to human relationships. There are many relationship categories. Our emphasis is on risks associated with those you care about most.

Relationship risks include:

- Damaging relationships
- Losing relationships

Many factors can also affect wealth.

Wealth risks include:

- Diminishing or eliminating your ability to earn.
- Increasing your ability to spend your assets.

"Other risks" is a category that allows you to add to the list.

As you can see, your fitness condition can have a big impact on many areas you may not have thought about before.

These risks increase in proportion to your fitness level and the length of time you are out of shape.

**NOTE: The GOOD NEWS is that these risks can also be mitigated or eliminated very quickly. It is never too late -The benefits of improved fitness have been shown to reduce risks quickly regardless of gender, age, or length of time out of shape!**

Later on, we will help you consider your risks along these three quality of life aspects. Next, we will spend significant time covering information related to the health risks aspect. This is critical information and we hope you will spend the time going over it!

Health Risk

The National Weight Control Registry is a research study that seeks to gather information from people who have successfully lost weight and kept it off for a reasonable period. To be a participant of the study, a person must be over eighteen years of age, must have lost at least thirty pounds, and should have kept them off for a period of one year or more. As of the end of 2010, the average weight loss of the over 5000 participants was sixty-six pounds and they had kept the weight off five and a half years, according to information posted on their Web site. Those are impressive results!

One of the key findings of this study indicates that just over three quarters of the participants reported a "triggering" event prior to success. Unfortunately, that means that something significant happened that really shook them up and got them to see their fitness improvement efforts through to success. The "event," assumed to have been a negative experience in most if not all cases, finally got their attention for good. The significance of this point is that most in the study had attempted to get in shape more than five times prior to success in getting and staying in better shape. Thus, what we would like to accomplish is to prevent you from experiencing a real event that will trigger your ultimate success.

Thus, the goal of this particular section is to create a virtual event for you. We want you to use your memory and/or imagination to elicit the same strong, powerful emotions as a real triggering event would. Our aim with this section is to scare you as much as we can. However, please know that we are doing so with the best of intentions. The risks associated with poor fitness conditions are very real! We hope you get it and that we are effective in our goal to get you scared enough to energize your effort through success.

The Virtual Event

The question is do you wait until an event comes along in the near or far future or do you act NOW! If you determine your risk is worthy of action, the time to act is now not when a real event gets you going. If not now-when?-DO NOT WAIT!-It will be your choice to make. We will guide you through the process of understanding what can happen and feeling as close to the emotions as you would if it were the case. We realize this is a big challenge, perhaps the biggest one for all of us. Now that we have set the goal and purpose clearly, the next step is to get you educated with important and relevant information regarding poor fitness risks.

Key Risk Factors

Your current fitness level is the result of many interrelated factors. Outside any genetic or health-related condition, your fitness level is the result of a caloric intake imbalance. This means you are consuming more calories than those you are using in a typical day. Many of us eat too much "bad" food and do little or no exercise. For every 3,500 or so calories we intake above those we require, (around 1,800 for women and 2000 per day for men) we gain a pound of weight. In addition, for every five pounds we gain, we add around an inch or so to our waist. Furthermore, lack of exercise increases the amount of fat in our body and reduces the amount of muscle mass. Unused muscles shrink and excess calories are stored as fat for future use in the body. Fat around the belly has been found to be the worst kind from a health risk standpoint.

While there are several risk factors such as our genes and hazard exposures involved in determining risk, there are several key risks health professionals consider when assessing health and quality of life risks. First, is the body mass index and second is waist circumference.

The BMI

Body mass index, better known as BMI, is a measure of body fat based on height and weight that applies to adult men and women. It is a useful measure of overweight and obesity. Your height and weight are used to calculate it. BMI is an estimate of body fat and a good gauge of your risk for diseases that can occur with more body fat.

The higher the BMI, the higher your risk for certain diseases such as heart disease, high blood pressure, type 2 diabetes, gallstones, breathing problems, and certain cancers. However, since muscle is heavier than fat, BMI can overestimate body fat in cases of individuals who have a higher muscle mass than usual such as younger, active, or athletic people. Moreover, it can underestimate body fat in cases of those who have lower muscle mass such as older, less active, or less athletic people.

The table on the following page shows the heights and weights and the resulting BMI value.

If you prefer to view a larger copy, you may download it from www.fitnessprotocols.com/book/forms.pdf.

| Height | NORMAL RANGE | | | | | | OVERWEIGHT RANGE | | | | | OBESE RANGE | | | | | | | | | | |
|---|---|---|---|---|---|---|---|---|---|---|---|---|---|---|---|---|---|---|---|---|---|
| 58 | 91 | 96 | 100 | 105 | 110 | 115 | 119 | 124 | 129 | 134 | 138 | 143 | 148 | 153 | 158 | 162 | 167 | 172 | 177 | 181 | 186 |
| 59 | 94 | 99 | 104 | 109 | 114 | 119 | 124 | 128 | 133 | 138 | 143 | 148 | 153 | 158 | 163 | 168 | 173 | 178 | 183 | 188 | 193 |
| 60 | 97 | 102 | 107 | 112 | 118 | 123 | 128 | 133 | 138 | 143 | 148 | 153 | 158 | 163 | 168 | 174 | 179 | 184 | 189 | 194 | 199 |
| 61 | 100 | 106 | 111 | 116 | 122 | 127 | 132 | 137 | 143 | 148 | 153 | 158 | 164 | 169 | 174 | 180 | 185 | 190 | 195 | 201 | 206 |
| 62 | 104 | 109 | 115 | 120 | 126 | 131 | 136 | 142 | 147 | 153 | 158 | 163 | 169 | 175 | 180 | 186 | 191 | 196 | 202 | 207 | 213 |
| 63 | 107 | 113 | 118 | 124 | 130 | 135 | 141 | 146 | 152 | 158 | 163 | 169 | 174 | 180 | 186 | 191 | 197 | 203 | 208 | 214 | 220 |
| 64 | 110 | 116 | 122 | 128 | 134 | 140 | 145 | 151 | 157 | 163 | 169 | 174 | 180 | 186 | 192 | 197 | 204 | 209 | 215 | 221 | 227 |
| 65 | 114 | 120 | 126 | 132 | 138 | 144 | 150 | 156 | 162 | 168 | 174 | 180 | 186 | 192 | 198 | 204 | 210 | 216 | 222 | 228 | 234 |
| 66 | 118 | 124 | 130 | 136 | 142 | 148 | 155 | 161 | 167 | 173 | 179 | 186 | 192 | 198 | 204 | 210 | 216 | 223 | 229 | 235 | 241 |
| 67 | 121 | 127 | 134 | 140 | 146 | 153 | 159 | 166 | 172 | 178 | 185 | 191 | 198 | 204 | 211 | 217 | 223 | 230 | 236 | 242 | 249 |
| 68 | 125 | 131 | 138 | 144 | 151 | 158 | 164 | 171 | 177 | 184 | 190 | 197 | 203 | 210 | 216 | 223 | 230 | 236 | 243 | 249 | 256 |
| 69 | 128 | 135 | 142 | 149 | 155 | 162 | 169 | 176 | 182 | 189 | 196 | 203 | 209 | 216 | 223 | 230 | 236 | 243 | 250 | 257 | 263 |
| 70 | 132 | 139 | 146 | 153 | 160 | 167 | 174 | 181 | 188 | 195 | 202 | 209 | 216 | 222 | 229 | 236 | 243 | 250 | 257 | 264 | 271 |
| 71 | 136 | 143 | 150 | 157 | 165 | 172 | 179 | 186 | 193 | 200 | 208 | 215 | 222 | 229 | 236 | 243 | 250 | 257 | 265 | 272 | 279 |
| 72 | 140 | 147 | 154 | 162 | 169 | 177 | 184 | 191 | 199 | 206 | 213 | 221 | 228 | 235 | 242 | 250 | 258 | 265 | 272 | 279 | 287 |
| 73 | 144 | 151 | 159 | 166 | 174 | 182 | 189 | 197 | 204 | 212 | 219 | 227 | 235 | 242 | 250 | 257 | 265 | 272 | 280 | 288 | 295 |
| 74 | 148 | 155 | 163 | 171 | 179 | 186 | 194 | 202 | 210 | 218 | 225 | 233 | 241 | 249 | 256 | 264 | 272 | 280 | 287 | 295 | 303 |
| 75 | 152 | 160 | 168 | 176 | 184 | 192 | 200 | 208 | 216 | 224 | 232 | 240 | 248 | 256 | 264 | 272 | 279 | 287 | 295 | 303 | 311 |
| 76 | 156 | 164 | 172 | 180 | 189 | 197 | 205 | 213 | 221 | 230 | 238 | 246 | 254 | 263 | 271 | 279 | 287 | 295 | 304 | 312 | 320 |
| BMI | 19 | 20 | 21 | 22 | 23 | 24 | 25 | 26 | 27 | 28 | 29 | 30 | 31 | 32 | 33 | 34 | 35 | 36 | 37 | 38 | 39 |

Waist Size

Waist circumference is a simple measurement of the diameter of our waist. Studies have found that the fat the body stores around the waist area is the most harmful type and that diameters beyond a certain dimension are indicators of risk for men and women. A waist size greater than forty inches in men, and thirty-five inches in women, increases their health risks.

Male and Female Risks

The tables on the following page are based on data from the National Institutes of Health and they illustrate risk levels for several adverse health conditions, according to the aforementioned factors for both men and women.

## Men's Risk Level for type 2 diabetes, high blood pressure, and cardiovascular decease

| Condition | BMI (kg/m | For waist size equal 40 in or less | For waist size greater than 40 in |
|---|---|---|---|
| Underweight | Less than 18.5 | | |
| Normal | 18.5 to 24.5 | | |
| Overweight | 25.0 to 29.9 | Increased | High |
| Obese I | 30.0 to 34.9 | High | Very High |
| Obese II | 35.0 to 39.9 | Very High | Very High |
| Obese III | Greater than 40.0 | Extremely High | Extremely High |

## Women Risk Level for type 2 diabetes, high blood pressure, and cardiovascular decease

| Condition | BMI | Waist Size equal 35 in or less | Waist Size greater than 35 in |
|---|---|---|---|
| Underweight | Less than 18.5 | | |
| Normal | 18.5 to 24.5 | | |
| Overweight | 25.0 to 29.9 | Increased | High |
| Obese I | 30.0 to 34.9 | High | Very High |
| Obese II | 35.0 to 39.9 | Very High | Very High |
| Obese III | Greater than 40.0 | Extremely High | Extremely High |

**NOTE: Increased waist circumference also can be a marker for increased risk, even in persons of normal weight. Disease risk is relative to normal weight and waist circumference.**

As you can see, individuals with high BMI levels and/or large waist sizes are at ever-increasing risk of one or more adverse medical conditions not to mention significant degradation in the quality of their life as a result.

The figure that follows shows a generalized scale of risk. Please note that actual risks vary with each individual and his or her conditions and circumstances. Nonetheless, the higher our BMI and the longer it has been high, the higher the risks, and the worse the potential implications.

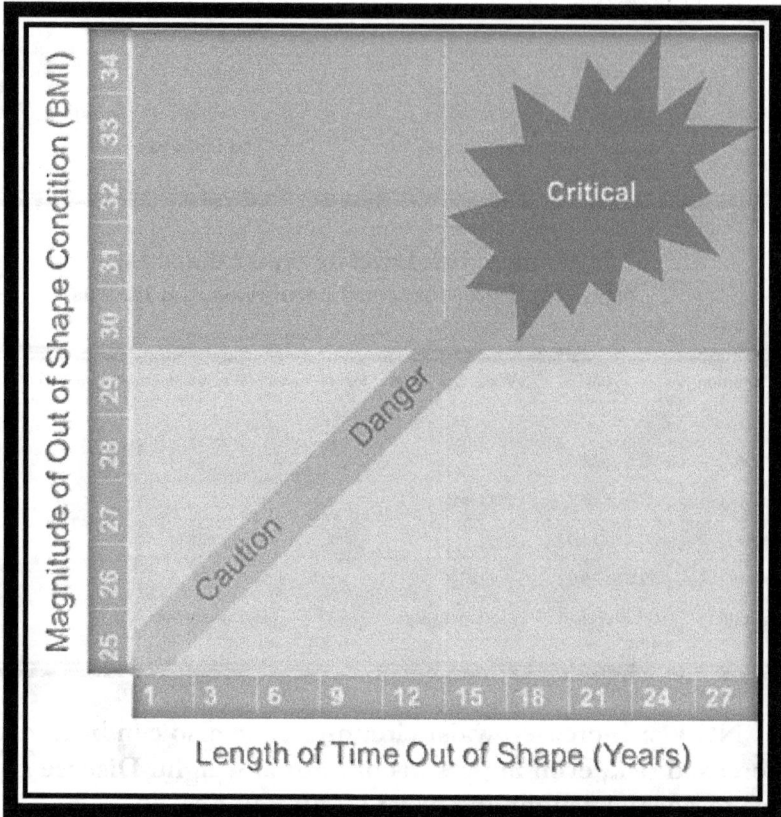

The following is a list of medical conditions that result from poor fitness:

- **Type 2 diabetes**
- **Coronary heart disease and stroke**
- **Metabolic syndrome**
- **Certain types of cancer**
- **Sleep apnea**
- **Osteoarthritis**
- **Gallbladder disease**
- **Fatty liver disease**
- **Pregnancy complication**
- **Reproductive issues**
- **Pulmonary problems**
- **High blood pressure**
- **High cholesterol**

If you have any doubts about these health risks, just visit a local emergency room anytime. Go to a hospital and walk around the hallways. Go visit some folks in a senior home and ask them how they feel. A poor fitness level will have a NEGATIVE effect on you and others you care about eventually! In the short term, it will make life less pleasurable. In the longer term, the ensuing physical discomfort, pain, and strain caused by such conditions are beyond what you can imagine, not to mention the emotional implications related to such situations. You can (and should) do something and the sooner the better. In addition to the reduction of health risks, better fitness can enable a much higher quality of life!

Relationship Risks

The two main risks involving relationships are the risks of damaging or losing them. Relationships are complex social phenomena and many factors influence their condition. Fitness condition has an effect on our relationships at many levels. It affects how we view others and how others see us. Our fitness influences who and how we relate. Our fitness affects our mood and our mood effects how we deal with others. Our fitness level determines the amount and quality of effort we can put forth and that, in turn, can affect how others feel about our ability to help or contribute to a group, family, or team. As our fitness deteriorates, we may find ourselves rejected or being distanced by others. Our ability to keep up socially or in sports may be diminished. The way others look at us or the comments they may make can affect the relationship.

Wealth Risk

Your fitness can have a significant impact on your wealth. The two main risks involving wealth and fitness are the risk of diminishing or eliminating your ability to earn and/or increasing your ability to spend your assets. Your ability to earn money is connected to your fitness level. A study conducted a few years ago by the State of New York Department of Education showed that fit students tend to get better grades and better jobs and end up earning more. The extent of your out-of-shape condition determines how you look and feel and it affects your energy, strength, flexibility, mental agility, and many other aspects important to wealth-producing activities whether we do physical work or knowledge work. Moreover, our fitness level also can affect how we spend. If your fitness level is poor, it may precipitate medical conditions and illnesses that require additional expenses in the form of fees or medications. In addition, less fit people are more prone to injuries and accidents, and it usually takes them longer to recover from such situations. As you can see, your fitness can have a big impact on your financial situation.

Short-Term vs. Long-Term Risk Considerations

Most of us live oblivious to the risk involved by being out of shape. As you have seen, the more out shape you are the higher the risk and the worst the potential implications can be. Unfortunately, most humans have a hard time getting motivation to solve problems that are not in the very near term. This means using these mostly longer-term implications to motivate you to change may not be very effective. We are wired to pay most of our attention to what is happening now or in the near term. It is a basic survival instinct. The reason for this is that our brain's limited energy needs to be freed up to make sure we can react to eminent danger. The "good news" is that there are enough short-term implications we can use to help make up for this.

Commitment

Short-Term Implications

As our shape gets worse, so does the quality of our life. Most of us do not do as well when we do not look and feel good. As our shape declines, it affects the way we look and feel. Our esteem and mood are affected. However, after a while, we can grow accustomed, and the longer we have been out of shape, the harder it may be to realize how good it used to be or it can be.

Beyond the impact on our health, our fitness condition affects the way we feel mentally and physically, which in turn affects our relationships and wealth directly or indirectly. Every point of BMI and/or inch on our waist have short-term implications: the image we see on the mirror gets bigger, the way others see and treat us changes, clothing does not fit as well, our energy declines, and the ability to move and do even simple and basic chores takes a lot more out of us.

Our fitness level can have a significant and nearly immediate negative or positive impact depending on which direction you are going. You can forget about the health risks for now; think about the quality of your life, about your ability to feel good, to have energy, strength, flexibility, stamina. That is the BIGGEST ticket! It is about the joy of life for us and for those we truly care about. It is real and it is NOW!

According to the 2009 Annual Medical Spending Attributable to Obesity by Finkelstein, Trogdon, Cohen, and Dietz, on average, people who are considered obese pay 42 percent more in health care costs than normal weight individuals.

According to the Yale University Rudd Center for Food Policy and Obesity:

*Obese people are highly stigmatized in our society; they suffer from inequalities in employment, education, and health care due to weight discrimination. Studies show that the media is an especially pervasive source of stigmatization against obese persons. A recent Rudd Center study found that 72 percent of photographs paired with online news stories about obesity are stigmatizing toward obese individuals. News photographs tend to portray obese individuals from unflattering angles (e.g., with only their abdomens or lower bodies shown) and engaging in stereotypical behaviors (e.g.,*

49

*eating unhealthy foods). These images degrade and dehumanize obese individuals, while spreading false assumptions and oversimplifying the complex issue of obesity.*

*In addition to suffering emotional and social consequences, obese individuals face economic disadvantages as a result of weight bias. The costs of weight stigma range from lower wages and fewer job and educational opportunities, to reduced access to quality health care.*

*The workplace is the most prevalent setting for weight discrimination. Overweight people may face biased hiring decisions even before they reach a job interview. Research shows that when a resume is accompanied by a picture or video, the overweight applicant is judged more negatively and is less likely to be hired. Promotion and firing are also influenced by weight discrimination. Research shows that employers see their overweight workers as poor role models; they describe overweight employees as lazy, sloppy, lacking in self-discipline, less competent and less conscientious. On average, obese individuals occupy lower-paying jobs and receive lower wages for the same jobs than their normal-weight counterparts. Women in the workplace bear a disproportionate amount of this impact.*

*Our society emphasizes physical appearance for both men and women. Such messages make overweight people feel unattractive. Many people think that obese individuals are gluttonous, lazy, or both, even though this is not true.*

*Emotional suffering can be the most painful part of being out of shape. People who are out of shape often face prejudice or discrimination in the job market, at school, and in social situations. Feelings of rejection, shame, and depression can be common.*

If you have been overweight or obese for even a short period, you have experienced at least one if not most of these effects. Moreover, while after some time some of us may become numb (or oblivious) to some of that, it hurts more that you may realize. It can affect you every day. However, the good news is that you can easily change the situation and that you can feel amazing when you do! In addition, it can change fast, and doing it may be easier than you may think. That is what this process is all about! You have taken the first step by choosing this approach. If you follow along and try some of what we will propose, you will be on the other side of these negative feelings and consequences very soon. We guarantee it-In fact, we PROMISE you!

Risk Assessment

Now it is time to assess your own risks in each category. You will use the following form to identify your top risks in the short, medium, and long term for each Quality of Life Aspect category:

You need to think which, if any, of the health risks you are at most risk for each period:

- Illness
- Injury
- Death

You need to think which, if any, of the relationship risks you are at most risk for each period:

- Damaging a relationship
- Losing a relationship

You need to think which, if any, of the health risks you are at most risk for each period:

- Diminishing or eliminating your ability to earn.
- Increasing your ability to spend your assets.

Now that you have a much better sense of all the possible risks, use the form on the following page to assess your own top risks.

If you prefer a larger copy, you may download it from www.fitnessprotocols.com/book/forms.pdf.

**NOTE: The top risks with the shortest-term implications should get you attentions and provide you with additional impetus for action.**

| | Health Risks | | | Relationship Risks | | | Wealth Risks | | | Other Risks | | |
|---|---|---|---|---|---|---|---|---|---|---|---|---|
| | 1 | 2 | 3 | 1 | 2 | 3 | 1 | 2 | 3 | 1 | 2 | 3 |
| Strong chance of happening within the next year | | | | | | | | | | | | |
| Strong chance of happening in two to five years | | | | | | | | | | | | |
| Strong chance of happening in more than five years | | | | | | | | | | | | |

## Step 3 - Consequences

This step will help you consider the consequences of improving and not improving your fitness.

About Consequences

So far, we have covered the drawbacks and risks involved. Now we will cover the consequences, or the positive and negative aspects that can result from your decisions or actions. Other terms used to describe them include after effects, aftermath, and outcomes. There can be both intended and unintended consequences from decisions or actions. Thinking about, identifying, and evaluating potential consequences is very important in the process of making your decision and building motivational energy to pursue your effort.

In order to get a fuller picture, we are going to look at four key dimensions of a consequence:

- What will happen if you improve your fitness.
- What will happen if you do not improve your fitness.
- What will not happen if you do improve your fitness.
- What will not happen if you do not improve your fitness.

Exploring all four dimensions will provide a much clearer picture of what may happen, one way or the other. Moreover, you will explore each dimension in relationship to you and to each of the three quality of life factors covered in prior sections. To facilitate this seemingly complex task, we have developed two forms, one to identify what may happen and another to identify what may not happen.

The Method to Our Madness

Please keep in mind that we are working on a multilayered approach to building your motivation and developing a sustainable decision. It takes time and effort to do but it will be well worth it later on. As mentioned in the introduction, this is the most critical section. You will build your success upon its foundation. Take your time to make sure you feel the energy each of these exercises will elicit. It will pay off, big time!

Impact Assessment

Take a moment to think about and identify what may happen if you choose to improve your fitness or if you do not.

Use the form on the following page to capture your thoughts.

If you prefer a larger copy, you may download it from www.fitnessprotocols.com/book/forms.pdf.

| What may happen | | | |
| --- | --- | --- | --- |
| To You | To your health | To your Relationships | To your wealth |

| If you improve your fitness | 1 | | | | |
| | 2 | | | | |
| | 3 | | | | |
| If you don't improve your fitness | 1 | | | | |
| | 2 | | | | |
| | 3 | | | | |

Take another moment to think about and identifying what may not happen if you choose to improve your fitness or if you do not.

Use the form on the following page to capture your thoughts.

If you prefer a larger copy, you may download it from www.fitnessprotocols.com/book/forms.pdf.

| What may not *happen* | | To You | To your health | To your Relationships | To your wealth |
|---|---|---|---|---|---|
| If you *improve your* fitness | 1 | | | | |
| | 2 | | | | |
| | 3 | | | | |
| If you *don't improve* your fitness | 1 | | | | |
| | 2 | | | | |
| | 3 | | | | |

## Step 4 - Other Not Wanted

This step will help you identify any other things you may not want that we did not cover in the prior sections.

The form on the following page is design to help you explore and consider things you do not want, more of, less of, bad, or high. Look at the form and give some thought to other things we may not have covered that you do not want out of your current fitness condition. The idea is not to create a long comprehensive list of all these things. Rather, we want you to find a few "high-energy" items you can use to continue building your conviction. You may circle existing items on the list or write the ones you come up with. You may skip this form if you feel there is nothing on it that energizes you.

If you prefer a larger copy, you may download it from www.fitnessprotocols.com/book/forms.pdf.

## Things I don't want ANYMORE!

| I don't want any | I don't want any more | I don't want less | I don't want bad | I don't want high | | |
|---|---|---|---|---|---|---|
| Pain | Pain | Energy | Health | Cholesterol | | |
| Criticism | Health Bills | Money | Looks | Blood Pressure | | |
| Bad feelings | Doctor Visits | | Comments | Stress | | |
| Medications | Weight | | Sex | | | |
| Stress | | | Relationships | | | |
| Rejection | | | | | | |
| Discrimination | | | | | | |
| | | | | | | |
| | | | | | | |

## Step 5 - Possibilities

This step will help you imagine all that can be possible when you improve and maintain your fitness.

About Possibilities

Possibilities are the things you could accomplish given you had more of several of the key benefits that improved fitness should deliver. At the end of this section, you will complete an assessment that will help you think of all the possibilities and identify the top one for you. In the meantime, we will provide you with a comprehensive review of the significant benefits of better fitness. The idea is to look at fitness from a broader perspective so that you may know how enabling these benefits can be, how much better your life can be, and how quickly it can happen in relative terms.

All-around Great Benefits

Benefits are positive aspects also known as plusses or advantages. Like the drawbacks, but to a lesser extent, identifying and emphasizing them can also provide significant positive energy for change. Once again, as with drawbacks, the benefits of living with a fitness level that is closer to the one we need to meet the needs of our key roles in life are not always obvious to us. A number of factors determine our level of awareness of some or all of the benefits of better fitness. Similar to the factors that affect awareness of the drawbacks, the length of time you have been out of shape and the extent of the gap between your fitness level and the ideal one will help you forget how you felt when you were in better shape. If you have never been in the best shape possible, it may be even harder to imagine. Thus, later in the section we will rely a lot on both memory and imagination to help harness positive motivational energy needed for the journey. The next few paragraphs will help refresh your memory and feed your imagination in preparation for the exercise at the end.

The Fitness Effect

Improved fitness leads to many benefits. The following list shows some of the mental and emotional POSITIVE effects reported by people who become fit:

- Feeling a greater sense of well-being.
- Having a more positive outlook on life.
- Feeling a strong sense of accomplishment and pride.
- Becoming more attractive (to others).
- Feeling a stronger sense of self-respect and self-worth.
- Having others see you and treat you differently (typically better).
- Feeling in a much better mood for longer periods.

Moreover, improved fitness can result in one or more of the following key benefits:

- Increased physical and mental energy
- More muscular strength
- Improved physical flexibility
- Stronger cardiovascular endurance
- Enhanced physical agility

Some of these benefits can be felt quickly after an improvement effort is undertaken. Moreover, the further you improve, the better it feels! You do not need to wait until you reach your final fitness goal to reap the benefits.

Depending on your life-style, life roles, and the stage of life you are at, you will have different needs for each of these benefits. Regardless, it is highly likely several of the following "meta-benefits" (benefits of the benefits) will result for improved fitness:

- Lower risk of injury, illnesses, and pain.
- Less time, effort, and pain to accomplish things.
- Higher quantity and quality of output.
- More pleasure and comfort working and playing.
- Faster recovery from illnesses and injuries.

In the end, when all is said and done, there is one single, but yet powerful benefit of being fit: You just feel so much better when you are fit to meet your life's needs-and there is NO better feeling than that-NONE!

Better Quality of Life

Let us now further explore what can happen if you become more fit. As mentioned earlier, fitness affects the key aspects of your life's quality:

- Your (mental and physical) health
- Your relationships with yourself and others
- Your emotional and financial wealth

Improved fitness can result in a number of improvements within one or more of these aspects: better fitness enables you accomplish more, better, smarter, and within less time, possibly leading to an enhanced ability to make and/or save more money. It enables you to help others more, make more and better love, be less grumpy, and to have fewer arguments about this (fitness) and/or other related matters. Finally, it enables you to have a stronger immune system and reduced levels of bad stress, both of which can lead to living a better and longer life!

Benefits from Multiple Perspectives

To appreciate the benefits of fitness further, you can also view it from several perspectives and related situations:

- The Working perspective
- The Playing perspective
- The Anytime/Anywhere perspective

The Working perspective

At work, improved fitness can lead to a number of positive outcomes, depending on the type of work you do. If your work involves physical activity, you have already read some benefits. However if your work involves knowledge work, improved fitness can lead to better ability to pay attention and focus. These are two critical success factors in any type of knowledge work!

At home, improved fitness can also lead to a number of positive outcomes, depending on your conditions and circumstances. Many people have long lists of chores to do at home:

- Yard work
- Shopping
- Doing the lawn
- Doing laundry
- Cleaning home and car(s)
- Fixing things
- Gardening
- Etc.

You can do all of these chores faster and better and it will take a lot less out of you when you improve your fitness. This can save you time and money if you are paying someone to do things for you due to your physical condition.

### The Playing perspective

Improved fitness leads to positive outcomes in several playing situations:

- Having fun
- Playing sports
- Hobbies

### Having fun

There are many ways to have fun and relax with friends and loved ones:

- Playing physical games with family and friends.
- Dancing and making love.
- Etc.

Improved fitness provides tremendous benefits while you engage in any of these activities.

### Playing sports

Not only do sports benefit from improved fitness but also doing so reinforces your fitness level as long as you stay injury free! The following lists some of the most common sports people enjoy playing both formally and informally:

- Running
- Swimming
- Tennis
- Baseball
- Basketball
- Football
- Other

## Doing Hobbies

People engage in many different hobbies. Some require more physical effort than others do. Nevertheless, all hobbies can benefit from your improved fitness. No matter what hobby you enjoy, by improving your fitness you will most likely experience higher performance and enjoyment of your hobbies!

## The Anytime/Anywhere perspective

Last, but not least, improved fitness will make the most basic tasks and functions we do day to day and sometimes hour by hour a lot easier. The following things we do will benefit from better fitness:

- Sleeping
- Pushing and pulling things.
- Walking
- Climbing
- Bending down
- Standing up
- Carrying
- Lifting
- Driving
- Getting in and out, and on and off things.
- Sitting down and getting up.
- Getting dressed
- Remaining seated
- Fitting in seats and other tight spaces.
- Etc.

## Additional Fitness Benefits

There are additional benefits you should also consider. Certain injuries and illnesses benefit greatly from improved physical fitness. Individuals with knee problems, for example, can do much better with lower body weight. Running to become and remain fit improves a somewhat common condition known as plantar fasciitis. Moreover, losing weight, typically necessary to improve one's fitness level, improves, and sometimes cures, certain types of diabetes. Furthermore, cholesterol and blood pleasure levels improve with fitness, thus reducing other health risks associated with them.

In a 1986 study, Chodzko-Zajko and Ismail found that physical fitness was a significant discriminator between those who experienced depression and those who did not. The physically fit had a significantly lower risk of depression than did those with low levels of fitness. Moreover, those more physically fit are more likely to survive accidents and recover faster from injuries and illnesses.

Fitness is much more impactful than you think! Moreover, getting fit provides very quick benefits in many more areas you can imagine. It affects the quality of your life. Every five to ten pounds you shed has an impact. Every inch you lose has an impact. The positive impact can be felt soon after you undertake the effort to improve. You do not need to wait until next year, or five years from today.

Finally, fit people are able to become more "powerful" and "independent"-That means that they tend to depend a lot less on others for their living success.

Having more energy, strength, flexibility, endurance, and agility will have a lot more impact on the quality of your life (relationships, wealth, and heath) than you can imagine. It feels amazing when you achieve it and is thus well worth the effort! The possibilities are endless!

Possibility Assessment

Use the form on the following page to imagine possibilities. Think of what could be possible given the listed benefits. Once you complete your list, choose the top three possibilities by ranking their importance to you. Use a "1" to identify the most important one to you, a "2" for the next-most important, and so on. We are looking for the top five or so. Thus, there is no need to rank them all.

If you prefer a larger copy, you may download it from www.fitnessprotocols.com/book/forms.pdf.

| Fitness Benefits | | Imagine The Possibilities.... | The Most Important |
|---|---|---|---|
| If I had more Energy I could... | 1 | | |
| | 2 | | |
| | 3 | | |
| If I had more Strength I could... | 1 | | |
| | 2 | | |
| | 3 | | |
| If I had more Flexibility I could... | 1 | | |
| | 2 | | |
| | 3 | | |
| If I had more Endurance I could... | 1 | | |
| | 2 | | |
| | 3 | | |
| If I had more Agility I could... | 1 | | |
| | 2 | | |
| | 3 | | |
| If I looked better I could... | 1 | | |
| | 2 | | |
| | 3 | | |
| If I felt better I could... | 1 | | |
| | 2 | | |
| | 3 | | |

## Step 6 - Impact

This step will help you consider the impact of better fitness on your most important roles.

About Impact

The impact of the key benefits of improved fitness can be obtained quickly as you make progress toward your ultimate goal and can end up being significant to many of your key roles. Having more energy, strength, flexibility, etc. can affect how you do certain things and how much you enjoy them. Just imagine how much nicer it would be to do some of the most basic tasks and chores. Bending down to pick up after the kids or spouse (hubby) will take less effort. Even doing the laundry, cleaning the house, etc. will take so much less out of you.

Having more energy, strength, flexibility, endurance, and agility will have a lot more impact than you can imagine. Not to mention it can also reduce the time it takes you to do all of it, as you will be able to work faster because you are more fit and have more endurance. It will feel amazing when you achieve your improvement!

Impact Assessment

Use the form on the following page to think and identify a list of the top things each key benefit would enable you to do more, better, etc. for each of the key roles in your life. Please remember that we are looking to build you conviction. The idea is to identify the few most energizing items in each of these exercises. You need to feel emotional energy when you look at the top three or so, on these lists.

If you prefer a larger copy, you may download it from www.fitnessprotocols.com/book/forms.pdf.

## The Impact of Fitness Benefits on my Important Roles

| Benefits | | As Parent | As Spouse/Partner | As Daughter/Son | As Sister/Brother | As a Friend |
|---|---|---|---|---|---|---|
| More Energy would allow me to | 1 | | | | | |
| | 2 | | | | | |
| | 3 | | | | | |
| More Strength would allow me to | 1 | | | | | |
| | 2 | | | | | |
| | 3 | | | | | |
| More Flexibility would allow me to | 1 | | | | | |
| | 2 | | | | | |
| | 3 | | | | | |
| More Endurance would allow me to | 1 | | | | | |
| | 2 | | | | | |
| | 3 | | | | | |
| More Agility would allow me to | 1 | | | | | |
| | 2 | | | | | |
| | 3 | | | | | |

## Step 7 - Needs

This step will help you identify where your top fitness needs are.

About Fitness Needs

As mentioned several times before, we all have different fitness needs that vary according to what we must do or like to do. Your ideal fitness level or condition enables you to look and feel good while meeting the physical and mental demands required by the tasks of your most important life roles. In this case, we are allowing you to think of the needs for the key fitness benefits in the context of the three main locations you would normally require one or more of the fitness factors and key benefits.

Needs Assessment

Use the form on the following page to think about and identify where you could use more of each benefit, where you have enough, and where you may have more than you think you need.

If you prefer a larger copy, you may download it from www.fitnessprotocols.com/book/forms.pdf.

## Fitness Benefits Needs Assessment

| Key Fitness Benefits | Need/want More at | | | I Have Enough at | | | I Have Too Much at | | |
|---|---|---|---|---|---|---|---|---|---|
| | Home | Work | Play | Home | Work | Play | Home | Work | Play |
| Energy | | | | | | | | | |
| Strength | | | | | | | | | |
| Flexibility | | | | | | | | | |
| Endurance | | | | | | | | | |
| Agility | | | | | | | | | |

## Step 8 - Other Wanted

This step will help you identify any other things you want to get out of improving your fitness that we did not cover in the prior sections.

The form on the following page is design to help you explore and identify other things you want more of, less of, bad, or high. Look at the form and give some thought to other things we may not have covered that you want to get out of improved fitness. They idea is not to create a long comprehensive list of all these things. Rather, we want you to find a few "high-energy" items you can use to continue building your conviction. You may circle existing items on the list or write the ones you come up with.

You may choose to skip this form if you feel there is nothing on it that energizes you.

If you prefer a larger copy, you may download it from www.fitnessprotocols.com/book/forms.pdf.

## Things I want really BAD!

| I want more | I want better | I want larger | I want less | I want lower | I want smaller |
|---|---|---|---|---|---|
| Joy | Feelings | Income | Pain | Stress | Waist |
| Energy | Job | Muscles | Discomfort | Cholesterol | Belly |
| Stamina | Play | Business | | Harte rate | Butt |
| Flexibility | Health | | | | Legs |
| Sex | Looks | | | | Arms |
| Time | Sex | | | | |
| Fun | Sleep | | | | |
| Comfort | | | | | |
| | | | | | |

## Step 9 - Conviction Assurance

This step will help you ensure your level of conviction is sufficiently high to proceed.

The Importance of Strong Conviction

Your sense of conviction is a strong emotional feeling resulting from being highly convinced that you REALLY want to accomplish this task. Conviction results from the process of evaluating and building a strong rationale. In order to reduce or ideally eliminate any chance of relapse from one stage to another, or of even failing to accomplish your overall goal, you need to ensure you build the strongest possible case for better fitness. Without that feeling, your chance of success can diminish. Your energy can fizzle and you can be back where you started and sometime even worse off. You must want this very BADLY! Not one ounce of ambivalence must exist inside or anywhere near you. Your conviction is imperative!

The Key Aspects of Conviction

In this section, we will enable you to review the results from all the prior eight steps. In doing so, you can evaluate the rationale for improving your fitness and further enhance it if need be. This will be the first chance you have to look at the whole picture. You will see how it all comes together to make a strong case for taking the next step of preparing to take action.

The following image depicts the model we used to help you build your rationale.

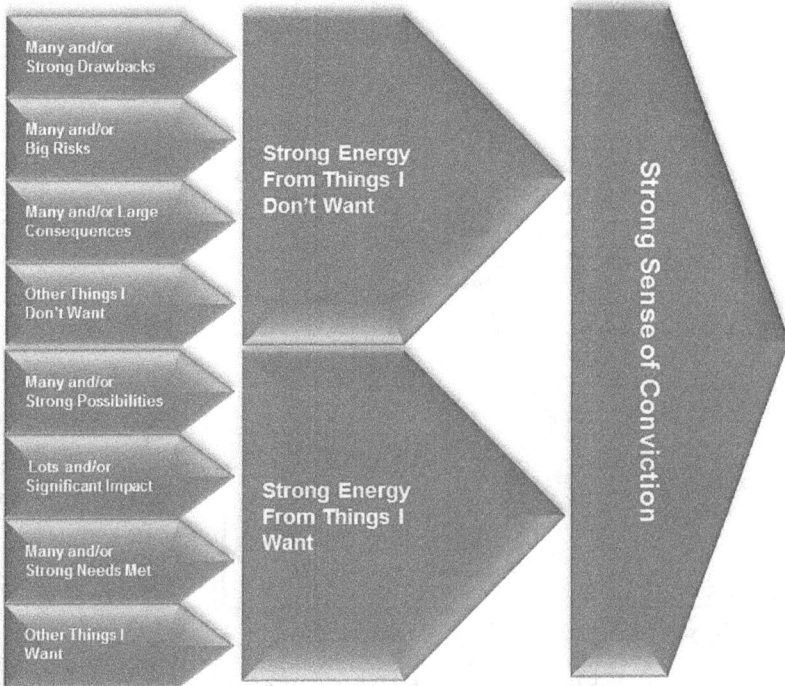

The Things You Don't Want

As mentioned earlier, your conviction depends on two key aspects: The things you do not want and those you do. Use the form on the following page to summarize all the things you really do not want out of your current fitness condition. Go back to the forms on page 35, 52, 55/57, and 59 and transfer the top three choices for each of the four areas listed into this form.

If you prefer a larger copy, you may download it from www.fitnessprotocols.com/book/forms.pdf.

# The Things I Really DON'T Want

## The Worst Drawbacks

## My Biggest Risks

## The Largest Consequences

## More Things I Don't Want

You should review the choices to make sure they reflect your feelings and they are truly the things you really DO NOT want! You MUST really HATE these aspects of your condition to produce part of the energy we need you to harness for the fullest conviction level we can muster out of you. Feel free to return to the respective section to review and edit any of them if necessary. You need to feel strongly about rejecting these from your life!

The Things You Want

Use the form on the following page to summarize all the things you really want badly from an improved fitness condition. Go back to the forms on page 67, 69, 71, and 73 and transfer the top three choices for each of the four areas listed into this form.

If you prefer a larger copy, you may download it from www.fitnessprotocols.com/ forms/wants_form.pdf.

# The Things I Want BADLY!

## The Strongest Possibilities

## The Most Significant Impact

## My Biggest Needs

## More Things I Want

You should also review these choices to make sure they reflect your feelings and truly reflect the things you want BADLY! You MUST really WANT these aspects BADLY in order for them to produce the second part of the powerful energy we need you to harness for the fullest conviction level we can muster out of you. Feel free to return to the respective section to review and edit any of them if necessary. You need to feel strongly about wanting these in your life!

The Conviction Rationale

At this point, the rationale for moving forward should be very clear to you! You should feel strongly about the impact that improving your fitness will have on your life in both the short and long run. The feeling you are looking for is one where come hell or high water—no matter what comes your way—you will improve your fitness. That you will do whatever it takes and accomplish your goal. Moreover, nothing and no one will get in the way of your effort. It needs to be that clear and feel that strong inside you. You should not feel one ounce of ambivalence or doubt about this. This is your main energy source and you must revisit it occasionally when the going gets tough. You need to keep your reasons present at all times to remind you why you are doing this.

Are you ready? Do you have enough conviction to get going and stay with it? If the answer is yes, move on to the next step. If not, feel free to revisit the process. Spend more time and dig deeper for those things that you care most about; make the strongest possible connection to improving you fitness.

**NOTE: This is the most critical step of the process. We highly recommend you do not proceed further until your conviction is very high!**

## The Formal Commitment

This part will help your formalize and document your commitment to improve and maintain your fitness.

Your Commitment is Critical

As we mentioned in the introduction, commitment is a critical success factor in this process. It is critical because it is what powers your determination and that is what will ultimately see you though all stages of the Fitness Protocols™.

The Dynamics of Commitment

By this point, you should have already built both a strong sense of readiness for the effort and a strong sense of conviction based on a solid rationale for better fitness. The dynamics of your commitment should have shifted and you should feel highly confident about what you want to accomplish. The following diagram shows the "new" dynamic image.

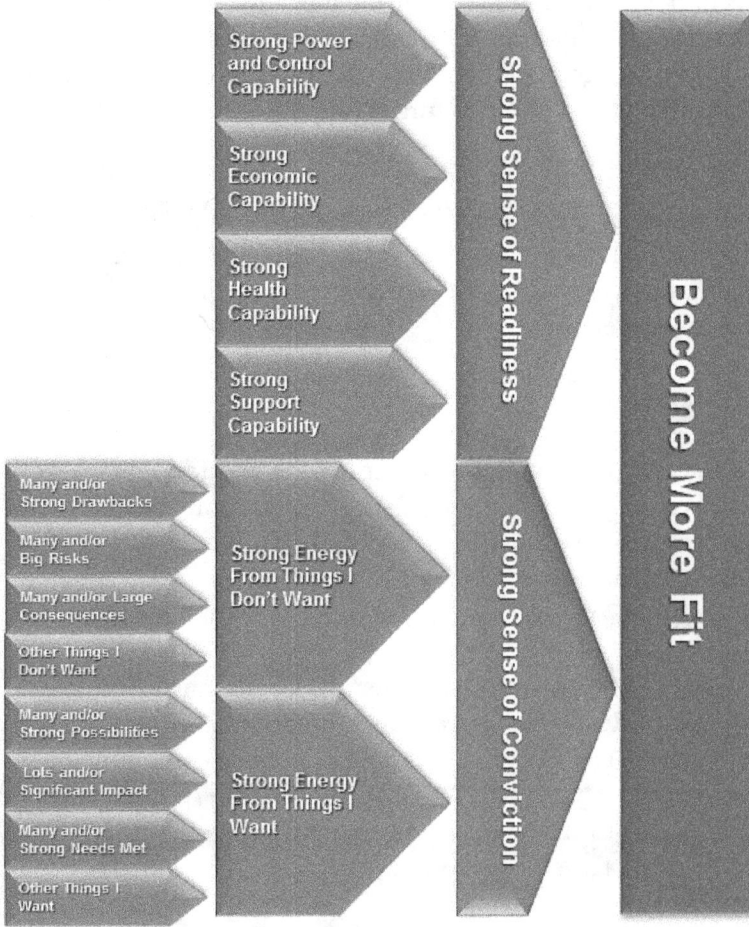

In this new dynamic, you should feel a strong sense of readiness supported by a strong sense of power and control, economic, health, and support capabilities. Moreover, a strong sense of conviction supported by a strong sense of the things you do not want and those you do. That is the image you must have in your mind and feel in your emotions.

Any doubts that may linger are normal and most likely relate to the fact that you lack a full sense of what you need to do to accomplish your goal at this point. However, the good news is that that is what the next step is going to be. In the next preparation stage, we will get you ready with the knowledge and skills you will need to be successful. If for any reason doubts regarding any of the items on the commitment model are still not fully energized, feel free and comfortable to go back to revisit them—There is nothing wrong with that. It is critical you get both strong senses! By the way, you can return at any time in the process if doubts emerge. It is OK!

Assuming all is fine and you are ready to take the plunge, please complete the following final step. This step is the formal commitment statement. Here you will sign a formal statement of commitment to your goal and ensuing effort.

If not now—when?

The time has come to commit to look and feel much better!—To have more energy!—To be stronger!—To be more flexible!—To have more endurance!—To be able to get more things done!—And to enjoy your life with those you care most about, doing the things you love doing, and getting as much out of it as possible! The time is NOW.

You will find a form with the final commitment statement in the following page. Read it to make sure it reflects your true feelings. When you feel ready, date and sign it as a symbol of your commitment.

Feel free to make a copy and consider posting it in a prominent place to help you remember it often.

Alternatively, you can create your own commitment statement with words that reflect your feelings better.

If you prefer a larger copy, you may download it from www.fitnessprotocols.com/book/forms.pdf.

Congratulations on accomplishing this MOST critical phase! You should now be ready to move on to the preparation protocol where we will help you get ready to improve your fitness.

# My Commitment

I do hereby commit to undertake the effort to improve my fitness, and to maintain it at a level that is best suited to my wants and needs.

My commitment to do so is founded on a strong sense of readiness to undertake this effort, and on an unequivocal conviction that looking and feeling better will enable me to live a more productive, joyful, and fulfilling life.

This _____ Day of _____

_____
Signature

 *Fitness Protocols*™

# Preparation

This protocol will help you prepare to improve your fitness.

About Preparation

Preparation is the second stage in the overall process as shown in the figure below. Improving fitness typically requires a change in approach. Preparation involves the effort to get you ready to change your fitness approach successfully.

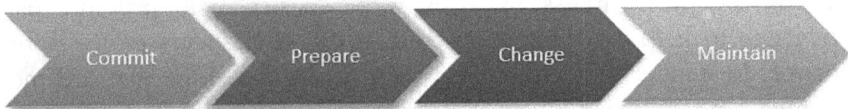

This stage is very important because preparation should increase your confidence. When you add confidence to your determination, the chances of your success should be much higher. Moreover, feeling better prepared should make accomplishing the goal seem much easier. Besides the new knowledge and confidence you will gain during this stage, you will also develop a set of plans to help guide and support your improvement effort.

Further substantiating the importance of this section, a study conducted by Dholakia, Bagozzi, and Gopinath, published in the February 2007 edition of the online Journal of Behavioral Decision Making, showed how remembering past actions and formulating implementation plans can facilitate enactment of effortful decision. People with a plan tend to do much better at achieving their goals than those without one. If you want to succeed at anything, you have to prepare and plan accordingly. You need to take the time to do it. That is exactly what this section is all for.

The Process of Preparation

The following figure shows the main preparation sections you should cover in this section.

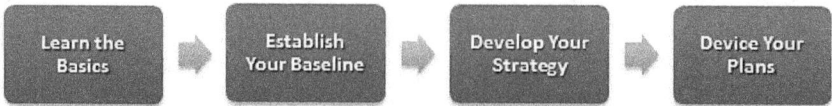

Learning the Basics

Lack of awareness and knowledge is one of the negative factors affecting people's fitness. Learning the basics will provide basic knowledge to help you better understand the key aspects of the fitness dynamic. Moreover, it will enable you to make decisions that are more informed, and devise a more comprehensive approach to your fitness. Once equipped with the basics, you will move on to the next section where you will establish your baseline or starting point.

Establish Your Baseline

In order to develop appropriate goals and plans to accomplish them more effectively, you need to know where you are now. Your baseline is simply the set of facts regarding your current fitness situation. This information will help better scope your effort and feed the process that determines the best strategies to help you realize and achieve your improvement goals.

Develop Your Strategy

Your strategy is the approach you will take to accomplish your goal. To develop your strategy you will consider your current situation together with its root causes from the baseline section. The strategy should move you from where you are to the goals you set by taking actions that address the root causes of your condition.

Devise Your Plans

Finally, you will develop a number of plans that will guide your effort to accomplish the individual goals set in the prior section, which together should lead to meeting your overall fitness improvement goal.

## Learn the Basics

This part will help you gain a good understanding of how key aspects of the human mind and body interact and affect fitness.

As the figure below illustrates, this is the first of four steps intended to help you learn the basics of fitness.

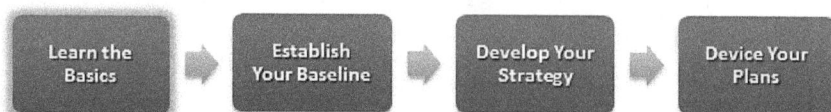

| Learn the Basics | → | Establish Your Baseline | → | Develop Your Strategy | → | Device Your Plans |

About the Fitness Dynamic

Your fitness condition is the result of a number of decisions and behaviors. The dynamic process originates and ends in the mind. However, the mind and the body are tightly connected and interrelated; thus, they cannot be separated per se.

A number of internal and external factors influence our decisions and the behaviors and actions that result. Understanding this dynamic is critical to your success. Therefore, we have developed a model to clarify how it works, which we refer to as the Fitness Dynamic Model™.

The model, shown in the next page describes the six key factors that influence what, when, where, and how much we eat and do. Our behavior leads to the level of nutrition, activity, and energy balance that results in how well we do, look, and feel on a daily basis.

Understanding how this dynamic works can make a big difference to you! Please make a concerted effort to understand it in the following two sections. Spend as much time as necessary to accomplish this objective.

We have broken up the "Learn the Basics" content into two sections: How the Mind Works and How the Body Works.

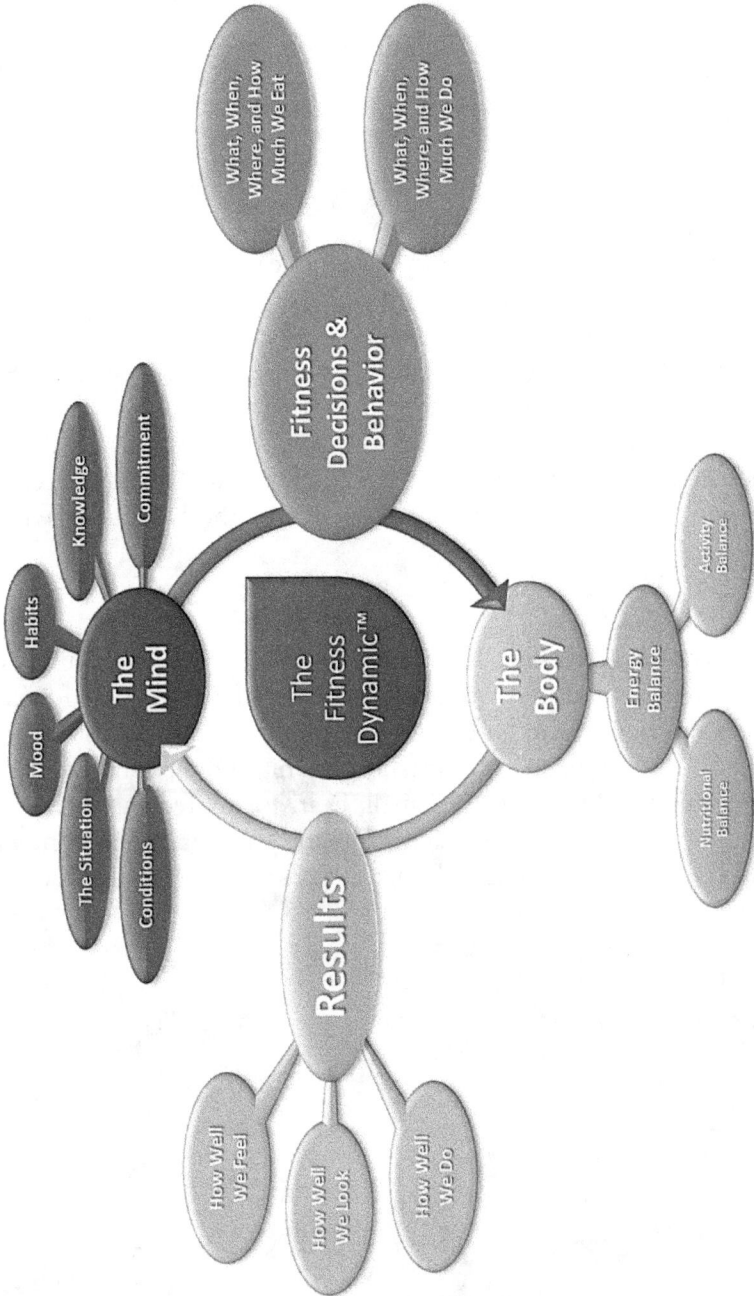

The Mind
— Knowledge
— Commitment
— Habits
— Mood
— The Situation
— Conditions

Fitness Decisions & Behavior
— What, When, Where, and How Much We Eat
— What, When, Where, and How Much We Do

The Fitness Dynamic™

The Body
— Activity Balance
— Energy Balance
— Nutritional Balance

Results
— How Well We Feel
— How Well We Look
— How Well We Do

## How the Mind Works

This part will help you understand the key aspects of the mind that affect fitness.

The Human Mind

The mind is an amazing, complex, and unique human capability. Our mind gives us the capacity to communicate with language, to think, and make decisions that lead to our behavior.

The mind resides inside the brain and is made of a bunch of highly structured and organized sets of brain cell connections. These structures are processed and stored in particular sections of the brain, depending on what they relate to. They are created from the electrical signals sent to the brain from our five senses via the nervous system.

How We Perceive

According to our understanding of the Neuro-linguistics and Neuro-Semantics theories, massive amounts of information constantly bombard the brain from all our senses during every conscious moment. Literally billions of bits of information are hitting our senses at any one moment. All the things we see, smell, hear, touch/feel, and think about in one moment can be overwhelming! To help us cope with so much, we have developed a set of "filters" that help chunk all that data down to a manageable size.

These mental, or perceptual filters, as they are better known, chunk down information by deleting portions of it, distorting it, and/or generalizing it as shown in the figure below.

Preparation

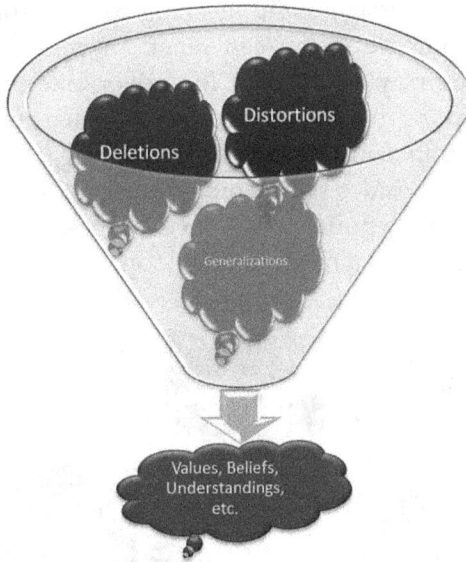

Our intentions, goals, etc. typically guide our attention, unless we have matters that are more critical, such as a threat to our life, or any other big attention-getting matter in front of us.

Accordingly, we may delete any information deemed not important. In other cases, we may distort information so it better fits the way we see things according to what we know, understand, value, believe, or hope. We will also generalize or draw conclusions from the data we get by quickly associating the input we get to a few prior experiences.

The brain is one busy entity and it needs to have as much of its "power" available as possible. So the faster it can process all this data, the faster it is free to process its next task. Most of this filtering and chunking happens fast, in the background, and we are not aware of it.

The Meaning of Meaning

This is how our fitness, and all other beliefs, values, understandings, and attitudes have come to be. It is how we end up assigning the meaning we give things. That meaning, in turn, produces the emotional energy that compels us to act or not to act.

Ultimately, we assign some meaning to everything. We have to. The level of meaning we assign can range anywhere from completely meaningless to extremely meaningful. Moreover, our emotional responses are directly proportional to the meaning assigned things. That is why things we consider amazing or awesome may trigger goose bumps. In addition, things we consider sad or nice can trigger corresponding tears. The following diagram captures a high-level overview of how the process flows. As you can see, it is a never-ending loop.

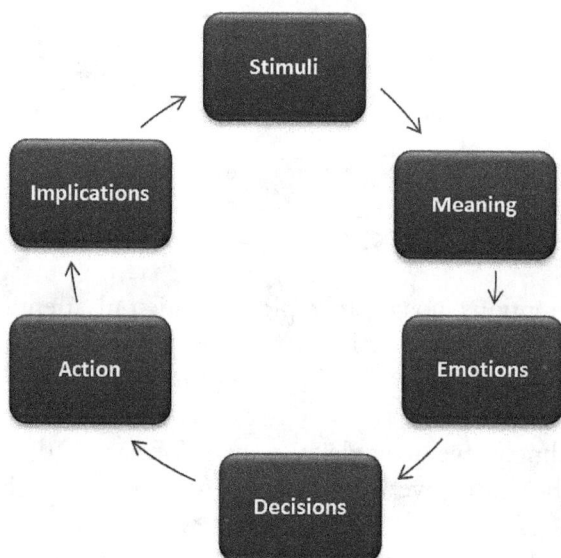

This process is how we end up making the decisions that lead to our behavior and the implications thereof. Implications are the feedback that lets us know if what we are doing worked for us. The process goes on.

The decisions that others and we made in the past have created the conditions we find ourselves in today. The food we chose to eat and amount of activity we expend determines, in large measure, our fitness level outside any genetic influences.

Now that you have a better understanding of how this complex process works, we can move on to examine six key fitness-related decisions and behavior factors shown in the next figure.

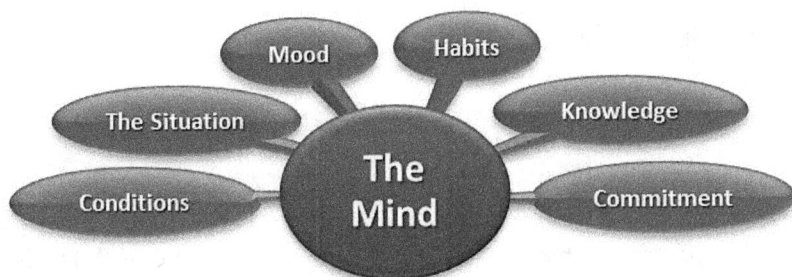

Following, we will describe each of the factors. We will explain how they influence your decisions and behavior. We will show how that leads to whatever level of nutrition, activity, and energy balance you have. In addition, we will show how it affects what you are able to do, and to how you look and feel.

Conditions

Conditions for this purpose are specific circumstances that can influence how we feel and therefore affect our fitness decisions and behavior.

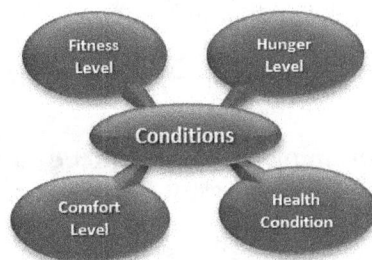

The figure above shows the four conditions we will cover in this section. Let us go over each one of them.

Fitness Level

Your overall fitness level affects you in many ways. In this context, it can influence how much you eat and do. The more out of shape you are, the bigger the challenge you can face. It can also affect how you feel both physically and mentally. Moreover, it can affect how others treat you, which, in turn, can affect how you feel. Your fitness level can be an influential factor!

Hunger Level

Your level of hunger can have a significant effect on you. The hungrier you are, the poorer your judgment can become. Hungry people are capable of doing almost anything in order to feed themselves. Eating is one of the most basic needs people must meet in order to survive. In your new approach to fitness, you must make an effort to avoid becoming too hungry by missing or skipping a meal or proper nutrients. It is not a good idea!

**NOTE: NEVER allow yourself to get too hungry-The hungrier you get, the worse the decisions you might end up making regarding food choices.**

Hungry people tend to eat more that those who are less hungry. Our animal instincts kick in and we will eat a lot of almost anything to satisfy this critical need.

Moreover, our ability to think and do things can also be compromised. Our attention fades from important matters, as the brain is missing critical fuel to function well.

**NOTE: Maintaining a well-balanced and consistent eating schedule is the best approach to follow.**

Health Condition

Your health condition can also affect your decisions and behavior. The impact this factor has depends on the type and severity of the condition. For example, injuries can prevent or limit activity and thus reduce your ability to burn calories. Other conditions may affect your appetite and influence what and how much you eat.

Comfort Level

Several environmental and ergonomic conditions can influence your level of comfort. Environmental factors include temperature, humidity, and the sounds and noise level where you find yourself at any decision point. Ergonomic factors relate to how comfortable a chair is and/or how high or low it is relative to a table.

As you can see, certain conditions can make a difference in what, when, where, and how much you eat and/or do. Therefore, you need to consider these conditions as you develop your new fitness approach.

The Situation

Certain situational aspects can be highly influential on our decisions and behaviors.

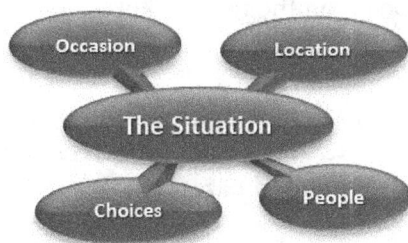

The figure above shows the four situational aspects we will cover in this section. Let us go over each of them.

Occasions

Occasions influence our judgment and behavior. Occasions include social events or situations like gatherings, meetings, luncheons, dinners, events, parties, etc. Most occasions come with food, drinks, and people. These three aspects alone can spell a challenge, never mind when you combine them all into one occasion. Alcoholic drinks can have an impact on our mood, judgment, and behavior. Food can abound in social settings. In addition, choices can be either limited or very wide, which can be a challenge either way. People in any setting can affect your mood, decisions, and behavior. Add drinks and food and the mix can get interesting and challenging, especially if you are just starting your new approach. Time spent in a social setting also takes you away from your set schedule and routines and that can present minor setbacks to your approach.

**NOTE: You may need to avoid some of them and carefully manage all others, especially early on. This could be one of your top challenges, depending on how much of a social person you are.**

Locations

Our location can have a big influence on what we decide and do regarding fitness. We can be at home, on the road in a car, visiting family or friends, out shopping in stores, or in a restaurant. Each of these locations can have different implications regarding our decisions and choices. Our location can affect the consistency of our fitness approach. Moving around and being on the road can present tremendous challenges to fitness efforts.

**NOTE: Our location and environment can affect our nutrition and the ability to be active. As with occasions, locations need to be considered and managed carefully.**

Choices

Having the right food and drinks available at the right time will be the hallmark of success. When those choices are not aligned with your approach and hunger sets in, you will eat anything available and thus can lose control of your approach, at least temporarily. This is another important aspect to manage!

**NOTE: Bad choices will lead to bad decisions. If this were to happen often enough, it could derail your effort.**

People

People can be highly influential on us, especially when it comes to nutrition and activity matters. The people we are with can make a big difference on a number of the key decisions regarding nutrition and activity. This is a critical consideration as you develop your new approach!

**NOTE: You need to surround yourself with people who understand, support, and respect your effort. Be leery of people who try to tempt you or attempt to sabotage the critical endeavor you are embarking on.**

As you can see, a number of these situational aspects can make a difference on what, when, where, and how much you eat and/or do. Therefore, you also need to consider them when you develop your new fitness approach.

Mood

Our mood is a highly influential factor on our decisions and behavior-perhaps the most influential!

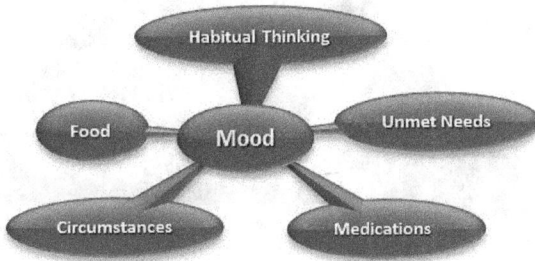

The figure above shows five factors that can affect how you feel, and therefore influence how you make decisions and behave. Let us go over each of them.

Habitual Thinking

Moods can habituate over time. The way we see people and things and whatever we feel about them produces positive or negative attitudes. These, in turn, become part of our habitual thinking patterns and can permeate our life, influencing our state of mind in positive or negative ways. We will cover more on this subject in the "Thinking

Habits" section later. Suffice it to say, our mood can be more a matter of habit than you can imagine. Your mood is yours and you have full control over it if you wish.

Unmet Needs

Unmet needs can have an unconscious impact on our mood. Let us take a minute to review some of the theory behind it. According to Abraham Maslow's theory of needs, human action is directed toward goal attainment. Around 1940, this now famous psychologist developed one of the most popular motivational theories known as "Maslow's Hierarchy of Needs." His theory often appears as a hierarchical pyramid model similar to the one shown below.

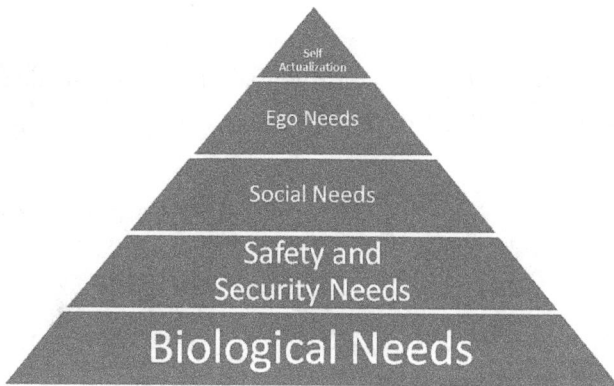

According to the theory, lower-level needs "must" be satisfied before the higher-level needs can influence decisions and behavior. However, any behavior could satisfy multiple needs at the same time.

- **Biological or physiological** needs are our most basic needs including the need for air, food, water, sex, sleep, etc.
- **Safety and security needs** include the need for a secure environment, ways to earn a living, good health, etc.
- **Social or belonging needs** include the need to belong, to love and be loved, and the need for friendship, intimacy, family, etc.

- **Ego or esteem needs** include the need to feel confident, self-esteem, achievement, respect, etc.
- **Self-Actualization needs** include the need to be creative, contribute, solve problems, express our talents, etc.

The first four levels are considered deficiency needs because, when not met, they drive us to meet them. Biological needs tend to be satisfied for most people, but when they are not, they become predominant. We will do almost anything to meet those needs! Emergencies or crisis safety needs also can rise to the forefront and become predominant. When our safety and security or that of others we care about is threatened, we can do amazing things! According to the theory, only after these first two need levels are satisfied can we be motivated to satisfy our social needs and then ego needs.

On the other hand, the need for self-actualization is not driven by deficiency per se. It is mostly driven by our desire for personal growth and the need to become all the things that we are capable of becoming, according to Maslow.

As you can imagine, or even experienced, any of the unmet needs can have a significant impact on our mood at any given time.

**NOTE: If you cannot find any obvious reasons to justify your mood, consider exploring the possibility that one or more unmet needs could unconsciously be the source of your state of mind. It can be very helpful!**

Medications

Both prescription and nonprescription medications can affect moods. In fact, that may be the purpose of some meds. In other cases, mood alteration may occur as a side effect of a particular med. Sometimes the same medication can affect the appetite.

**NOTE: Be aware and monitor how the medications can affect your fitness effort.**

**NOTE: Always consult your doctor or another credible medical authority before taking, changing, or stopping use of medications.**

Circumstances

Not many factors affect our mood more that our circumstances. Matters related to our health, relationships, and our finances are dynamic and can bear on us on a daily basis. Issues and problems we have can affect our mood.

**NOTE: Understanding how these factors affect you and finding ways to manage their impact can be of significant benefit.**

Food

The food we eat can affect our mood. Too much caffeine can make some of us hyperactive or cranky. Other food can have a soothing, calming effect. Too many of the wrong carbs can make us feel sleepy shortly after ingesting them. Alcoholic drinks have a significant and varying effect on people's moods.

**NOTE: It is important to know and understand how food and drinks we consume can affect us and affect our judgment and behavior.**

As you can see, many things can affect our mood. Moreover, our mood can greatly affect how we make decisions and behave. Mood awareness and management should be a key part of your new approach to fitness.

Habits

Habits are patterns of behavior learned and repeated until they become second nature. The force of habits can have a powerful influence on our life.

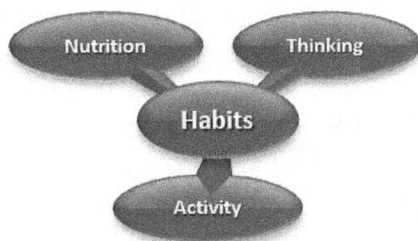

The figure above shows three habit categories we will expand upon in the following paragraphs. Habits are critical and they can represent the biggest challenges you will face as you attempt to improve your fitness. However, once you learn to conquer them, habits can become your best ally to keep your fitness approach in check possibly for the rest of your life. They are powerful!

As humans, we are creatures of habit. Our habits are thinking and acting patterns we develop over time through repetition and reinforcement. Habits evolve because our brain has limited capacity and "it" needs to keep as much of that capacity as free as possible. Therefore, as we learn things and practice them, we habituate them and they become things we do not think as much about. It is our nature to do so-The more we do things the more habitual they can become. Habits are literally wired in the brain's circuits, thus presenting us a potential challenge when we want to change them. Let us go over each one of the three habit categories shown in the figure above.

Thinking Habits

Our mood, as we mentioned earlier, can be habitual. Our personality is another form of habit. Personality is our unique way of being and it develops based on our own experiences and upbringing. Our attitudes can also be habitual. Attitudes are positive or negative ways of thinking about or looking at people and things. They are the mental constructs (beliefs) we develop over time. They represent your degree of like or dislike and can be positive or negative but can sometimes be conflicting like in those cases when you feel ambivalent.

Many attitudes are "inherited" or acquired from families or our cultures. In addition, that can sometimes make them challenging to change, especially the longer we have held them.

**NOTE: Your attitudes can play a big part in the process, especially those related to nutrition and exercise. Unchallenged attitudes can jeopardize your efforts. Make sure to examine all your attitudes; they can have a detrimental impact on your fitness effort.**

Activity Habits

What we do, when we do it, etc. can be habitual. Our physical activity patterns form over time. If you have been sitting down to watch TV, surfing the Web, etc. for a long time, it has most likely become a habit.

**NOTE: Your level and pattern of activity is most likely habitual. Changing it will be a challenge and should be done slowly. Do not try to start running marathons off the bat. Start slowly and build up.**

Consistency is more important than anything else is. Set a routine, follow it at the same time and of similar duration, and intensity-slowly build up from there. Your body will tell you when. At some point, you will not even need to be reminded, nor will you feel "forced to do it!- That is the power of habits!

Nutrition Habits

In addition, what we eat, when, where, etc. is most likely habitual. Moreover, usually the way we have been brought up has the biggest influence on our nutritional habits. We learn a lot by observing others, especially when we are young. Parents, family members, caretakers, and other influential people, at home and at school, have a big impact on our habits and us. Our eating patterns are nothing but programs in our brain that we can adjust and improve if necessary.

**NOTE: Knowledge and routines can help make the necessary adjustments. As with activity habits, setting an eating routine and schedule, and following it consistently, can be very beneficial to your effort.**

Knowledge

Knowledge is the accumulation of facts resulting from learning and experience.

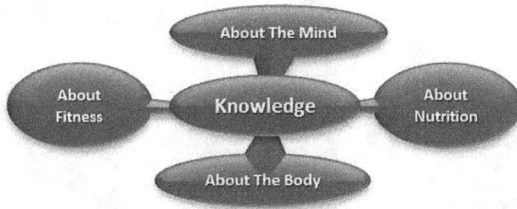

No matter what subject it is, the more you know, the better you should be. The right knowledge can be very powerful! On the other hand, the lack of it can be highly detrimental! The right knowledge can enable you to make better decisions and to behave differently. Knowledge provides a layer of power in addition to the power your commitment should provide. Knowing the right things provides additional energy to help overcome several of the challenges we have covered on this section. Ignorance is the enemy of fitness.

**NOTE: Learn as much as you can about how the mind works, the key facts about nutrition, the way the body works, and about fitness in general. That is what the "Learn the Basics" sections are for. They can make a big difference!**

Commitment

Commitment is a decision to stick with someone or something no matter what happens.

Earlier in the program, you spent significant time and effort building sustainable commitment to improving your fitness. The reason you did so is because the stronger your commitment is, the easier it should be to overcome the influence of your conditions, situations, habits, and moods.

Just to remind you, your commitment comes from developing and sustaining a strong sense of readiness and conviction, as the "house of commitment" figure shows below.

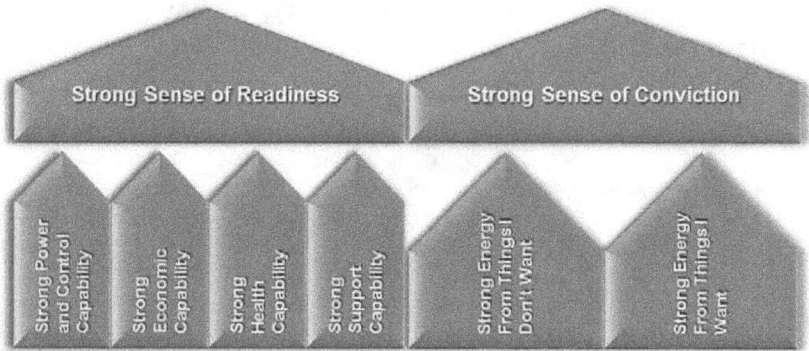

**NOTE: Feel free to go back to refresh your commitment occasionally in Section 1, if you feel it is necessary. You can never go wrong with that!**

Additional Energy and Power

You will be tempted and tested several times over as you move forward with your fitness improvement effort. Conditions, situations, moods, and habits will most likely push back on you often, especially early on, while you are implementing your new approach, and before new habits emerge and get set. Strong commitment and a solid foundation of knowledge can give you all the energy and power you need to overcome the power of these push backs.

The following figure illustrates how these forces work.

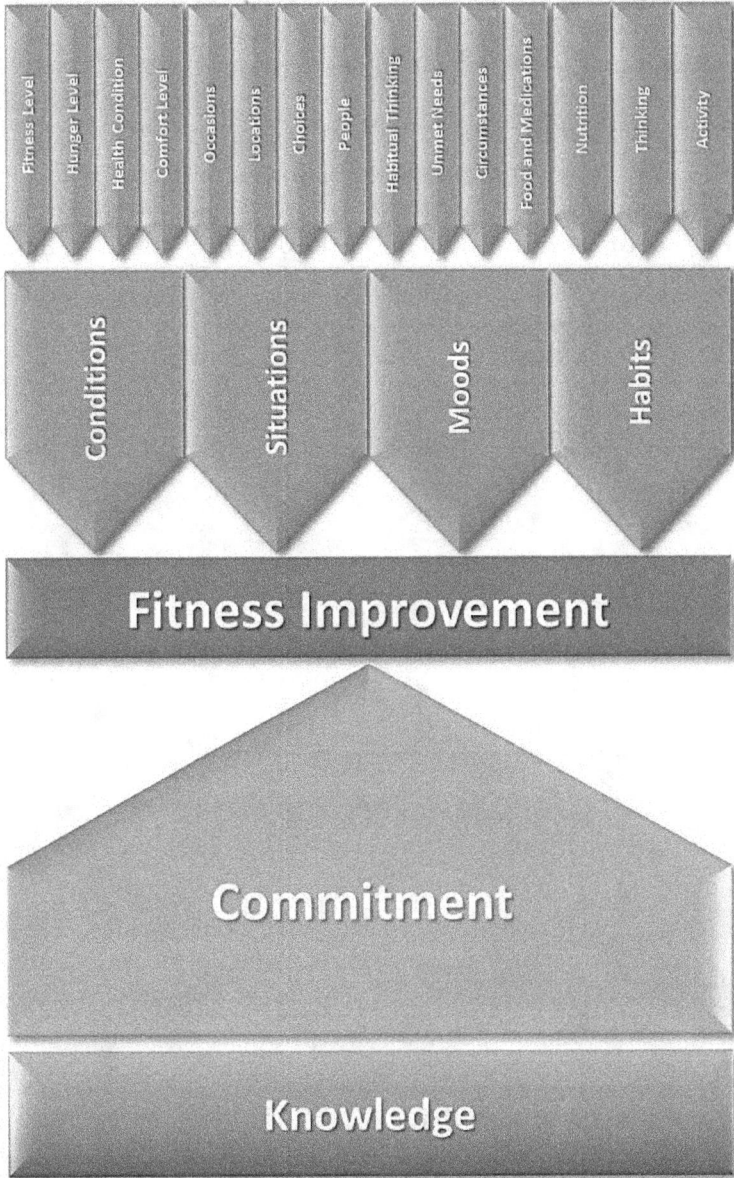

Fitness Level | Hunger Level | Health Condition | Comfort Level | Occasions | Locations | Choices | People | Habitual Thinking | Unmet Needs | Circumstances | Food and Medications | Nutrition | Thinking | Activity

**Conditions** | **Situations** | **Moods** | **Habits**

**Fitness Improvement**

**Commitment**

**Knowledge**

At any point, you can encounter one or several of sixteen push back aspects. Some will be harder to overcome than others will, but all will come your way at one point or another. The good news is that, sooner than you think, they will become less and less challenging. As you make progress and improve your fitness, you will get additional energy from that and habits will start forming. In turn, it will get much easier.

**NOTE: Conditions will change, situations will emerge, moods will swing, and habits may creep back here and there. However, your commitment and knowledge should help you prevail. Just keep at it-Never give up!**

## How the Body Works

This part will help you understand the key aspects of the body that affect fitness.

Your Body and Fitness

The body is amazing, complex, and complicated. It is composed of a number of incredible systems, which work independently and in unison to serve our human functioning. It is comprised of eleven major systems:

- Skeletal
- Muscular
- Nervous
- Skin, hair, and nails
- Lymphatic and immune
- Endocrine
- Cardiovascular
- Respiratory
- Digestive
- Urinary
- Reproductive

A fit body is one where all these systems are working optimally. Good fitness enables you to look and feel good. In addition, it makes meeting the physical and mental demands of your roles a lot easier to accomplish.

Physical fitness primarily involves five of the eleven systems on the list above:

- Skeletal
- Muscular
- Cardiovascular
- Respiratory
- Digestive

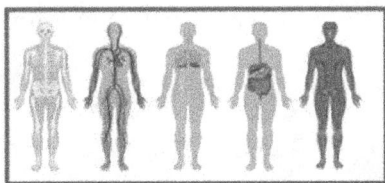

The appropriate combination of physical activity and nutrition can enhance and strengthen these systems according to the type, intensity, and frequency of activity expended, and to the type and quality of nutrients consumed. When these systems work better and are stronger, you can get one or several of the following benefits as a result:

- Increased physical and mental energy.
- More muscular strength.
- Improved physical flexibility.
- Stronger cardiovascular endurance.
- Enhanced physical agility.
- Better coordination.
- Better reaction time.
- Better balance.

Moreover, these benefits enable the following "higher level," or meta-benefits, as we called them earlier:

- Lower risk of injury, illnesses, and pain.
- Less time, effort, and pain to accomplish things.
- Higher quantity and quality of output.
- More pleasure and comfort working and playing.
- Fewer illnesses and injuries and/or faster recovery.

The Impact of Body on Mind

People who have achieved improved fitness report feeling a greater sense of well-being and having a more positive outlook on life. They feel a strong sense of accomplishment and pride when complimented for their fitness, or when accomplishing a task that was hard or impossible to accomplish prior. This leads some of them to feeling a stronger sense of self-respect and self-worth. Moreover, they feel others seem to treat them differently. All these positive aspects enable them to be in a better mood and remain in it for longer periods.

Three Balancing Acts

Good fitness is the result of a dynamic involving the three "balancing acts" of nutrition, activity, and energy.

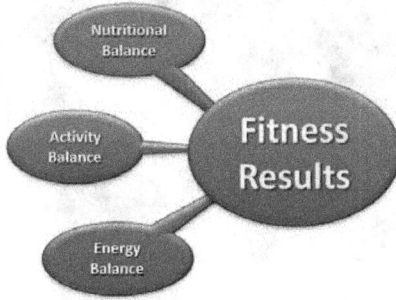

In this section we will help you understand how this dynamic works.

The figure on the following page describes the dynamic in detail. On the left side of the scale is the diagram showing the key aspects of nutritional balance. On the right side of the scale is the diagram showing the key aspects of activity balance.

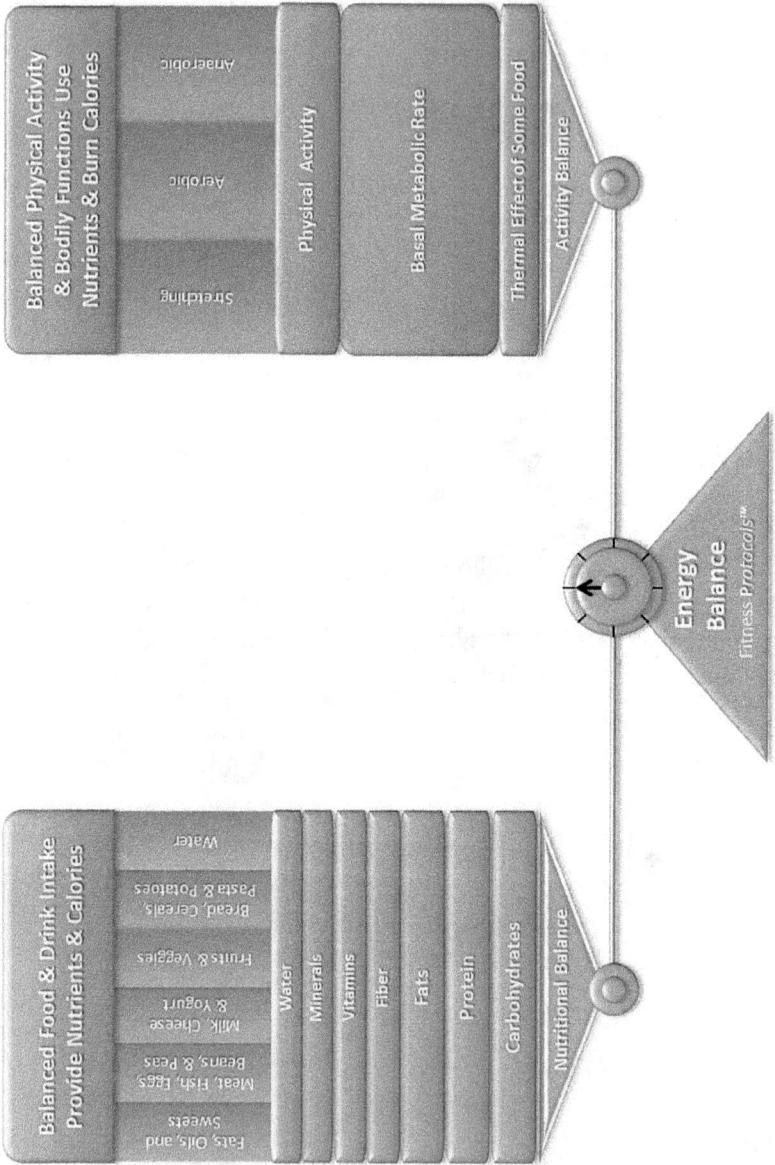

Balanced Physical Activity & Bodily Functions Use Nutrients & Burn Calories

Stretching | Aerobic | Anaerobic

Physical Activity

Basal Metabolic Rate

Thermal Effect of Some Food

Activity Balance

Energy Balance
Fitness Protocols™

Balanced Food & Drink Intake Provide Nutrients & Calories

Fats, Oils, and Sweets | Meat, Fish, Eggs, Beans, & Peas | Milk, Cheese & Yogurt | Fruits & Veggies | Bread, Cereals, Pasta & Potatoes | Water

Water | Minerals | Vitamins | Fiber | Fats | Protein | Carbohydrates

Nutritional Balance

Preparation

Following is a brief description of the three balancing acts.

Energy Balance

Balance seems to be a critical aspect in all of nature, and the human body is no exception. Energy or caloric balance occurs when the calories from the foods and drinks we consume are equal to the calories used or burned by the body as it functions and moves.

When calories consumed and burned are equal, our weight remains constant. However, we gain weight when more calories are consumed than those we burn, and we lose weight when we burn more calories than we consume.

**NOTE: For every 3,500 calories, one way or the other, one pound is added to or subtracted from the body's weight.**

The food and drinks we consume provide the energy and nutrients required to properly operate and move our body. Digestive and metabolic processes extract and/or convert the food you eat into the energy and nutrients we need.

Our bodies require a certain amount of energy, or calories, to conduct normal functions. The amount of calories each of us needs to be in balance varies according to a number of factors including gender, age, and level of activity. This number is known as basal metabolic rate or BMR.

The table in the following page shows the estimated number of calories required to maintain energy balance according to age, gender, and activity.

| Gender | Age (years) | Activity Level | | |
|--------|-------------|----------------|--------------------|--------|
| | | Sedentary | Moderately Active | Active |
| Child | 2-3 | 1,000 | 1,000 - 1,400 | 1,000 - 1,400 |
| Female | 4 - 8 | 1,200 | 1,400 - 1,600 | 1,400 - 1,800 |
| Female | 9-13 | 1,600 | 1,600 - 2,000 | 1,800 - 2,000 |
| Female | 14-18 | 1,800 | 2,000 | 2,400 |
| Female | 19-30 | 2,000 | 2,000 - 2,200 | 2,400 |
| Female | 31-50 | 1,800 | 2,000 | 2,200 |
| Female | 51+ | 1,600 | 1,800 | 2,000 - 2,200 |
| Male | 4-8 | 1,400 | 1,400 - 1,600 | 1,600 - 2,000 |
| Male | 9-13 | 1,800 | 1,800 - 2,200 | 2,000 - 2,600 |
| Male | 14-18 | 2,200 | 2,400 - 2,800 | 2,800 - 3,200 |
| Male | 19-30 | 2,400 | 2,600 - 2,800 | 3,000 |
| Male | 31-50 | 2,200 | 2,400 - 2,600 | 2,800 - 3,000 |
| Male | 51+ | 2,000 | 2,200 - 2,400 | 2,400 - 2,800 |

**Source: Dietary Guidelines for Americans: 2005**: These levels are based on Estimated Energy Requirements (EER) from the IOM Dietary Reference Intakes macronutrients report, 2002, calculated by gender, age, and activity level for reference-sized individuals. "Reference size," as determined by IOM, is based on median height and weight for ages up to age 18 years of age and median height and weight for that height to give a BMI of 21.5 for adult females and 22.5 for adult males. Sedentary means a lifestyle that includes only the light physical activity associated with typical day-to-day life. Moderately active means a lifestyle that includes physical activity equivalent to walking about 1.5 to 3 miles per day at 3 to 4 miles per hour, in addition to the light physical activity associated with typical day-to-day life. Active means a lifestyle that includes physical activity equivalent to walking more than 3 miles per day at 3 to 4 miles per hour, in addition to the light physical activity associated with typical day-to-day life. The calorie ranges shown are to accommodate needs of different ages within the group. For children and adolescents, more calories are needed at older ages. For adults, fewer calories are needed at older ages.

The thermal effect of food or TEF should be technically considered in the energy balance equation. Foods require energy to process or metabolize. Some foods require more energy for the amount they provide us. That means eating them actually ends up burning net calories without the need for any extra activity to do so. The grapefruit is one those foods that uses more energy to digest it that it provides. The TEF effect is usually low (less than 10 percent). Therefore, you should not be concerned about it too much.

Keep in mind that all key nutrients being protein, fat, and carbohydrates provide us energy. However, the body "prefers" energy from (good) carbohydrates. That is because it is more capable of using energy from carbohydrates than from protein and fats. Nevertheless, protein and fat have important functions.

The body will use them as an energy source only when it is does not get enough energy from carbohydrates. You will learn more about the basics of these and other important nutrients in the next section.

**NOTE: Study after study has consistently shown that Energy or Caloric Balance is the most critical factor when it comes to the weight management aspect of fitness. This means that you need to keep an eye on those calories!**

Nutritional Balance

Nutritional Balance is the dynamic involved in ingesting and properly digesting or metabolizing all the necessary nutrients from the food and drinks that we consume.

In order to maximize their full benefits we need to make sure we balance the type and amount of food we consume.

The figure below shows a model of the key elements involved.

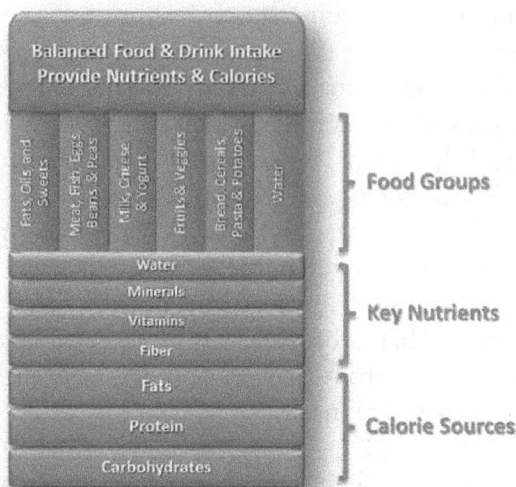

Following is a brief description of the key elements of this dynamic.

**NOTE: The best and most balanced approach to take is to eat meals with similar numbers of calories, which contain all the recommended amounts of nutrients. Moreover, we should eat at regular and consistent intervals throughout the day.**

The Metabolic Process

The foods we consume contain different amounts of energy or calories and different quantities and varieties of nutrients. Once ingested, the body metabolizes food to convert it into energy and nutrients for the body.

**NOTE: Any nutrients the body does not need when ingested, will either be stored for later use or get disposed of. Warning-Excess calories get stored (as fat) for later use.**

Preparation

The Essential Nutrients

The food and drinks we consume are made up of a combination of several of the following nutrients:

- Carbohydrates
- Fats
- Protein
- Vitamins
- Minerals
- Fiber
- Water

Following is a brief description of each of them.

Carbohydrates

Carbohydrates, or carbs, are also known as sugars or starches. They are one of the three essential nutrients we need to consume on a daily basis. Carbs exist in simple and complex form.

Simple Carbs

Simple carbs are considered "BAD" to consume because they raise blood sugar very fast and for a brief period as shown in the figure below. When blood sugar goes up that quickly, the body releases insulin to handle the excess. Insulin converts blood sugar into fat cells that then get stored in the body for later conversion back into energy in case the food we eat fails to provide enough at some point.

Another negative consequence of ingesting this type of carb is that it produces a quick rush of energy quickly followed by a foggy/lethargic or sleepy "out-of-it" feeling. Moreover, it induces hunger driving us to want to eat more.

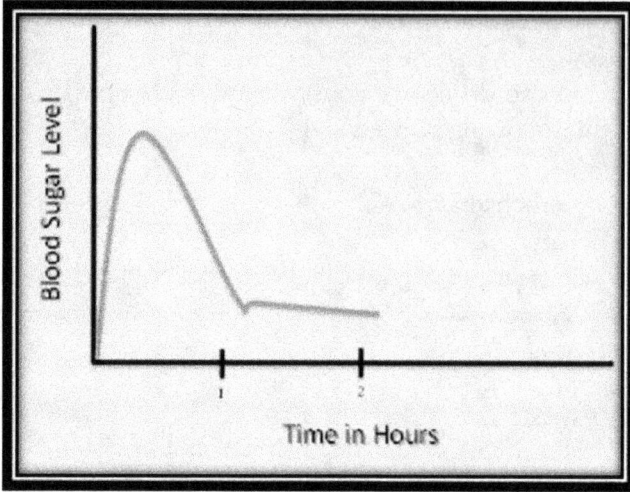

The following figure provides a list of some carbs to AVOID consuming.

## "BAD" Sugar Food & Drinks

| Sugar Food |
| --- |
| Table sugar |
| Corn syrup |
| Candy |
| Soda pop |
| Ice cream |

| White Flower Food |
| --- |
| Bread made with white flour |
| Pasta made with white flour |
| All baked goods made with white flour |
| Non-multi-grain packaged cereals |

Simple carbs are BAD for you under most circumstances and should be avoided unless you have a need for high energy very soon after you ingest them, as some athletes do. Otherwise, they will turn into fat cells that can quickly add weight if not burned. AVOID THEM!

Complex Carbs

Complex carbs are considered "GOOD," or better because they raise blood sugar at a much slower rate and to a lower level, as shown in the following figure. When blood sugar rises at a slower rate, insulin is not released. That means no fat is converted and stored. Moreover, they have a longer-lasting satiety effect when consumed and they do not cause the high/low effect that simple carbs create.

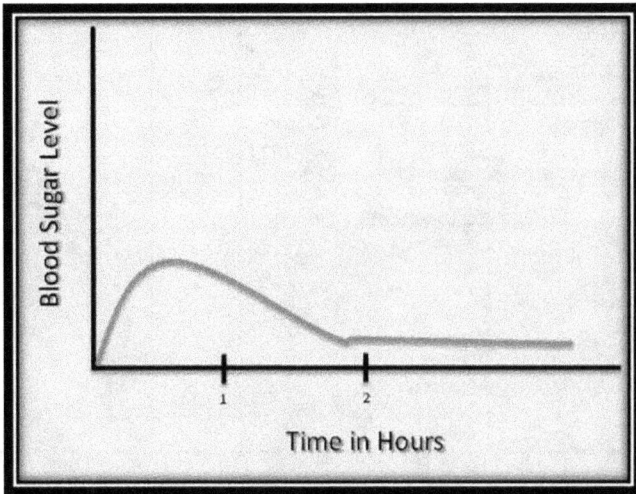

NOTE: You should seek to consume as many Complex Carbs as possible of your allowed daily carb consumption.

The following figure provides a list of carbs to consume.

## "GOOD" Carbohydrate-Rich Foods

| Potatoes | Rice | Pasta | Cereals | Breads |
|---|---|---|---|---|
| Yams<br>Sweet<br>Potatoes | Brown<br>Wild | Wheat | Oatmeal<br>Oat bran cereal<br>Museli<br>Whole Barley<br>Buckwheat | Multi-grain bread<br>Buckwheat bread<br>Oat bran bread |

| Seeds | Veggies | Fruits | Pulses |
|---|---|---|---|
| Soybeans<br>Garbanzo beans<br>Brussels Sprouts<br>Navy beans<br>Lentils<br>Split peas | Onions<br>Water Cress<br>Radishes<br>Okra<br>Carrots<br>Eggplant<br>Cauliflower<br>Cabbage<br>Broccoli<br>Spinach<br>Turnip Greens<br>Lettuce<br>Artichokes<br>Cucumbers<br>Asparagus<br>Zucchini<br>Celery | Dried Apricots<br>Plums<br>Oranges<br>Grapefruit<br>Strawberries<br>Prunes<br>Apples<br>Pears | Pinto beans<br>Kidney beans |

**NOTE: AVOID** Simple Carbs at all costs, unless you know you need the energy soon after consumption. These "BAD" carbs have become prolific in the food market and can be found everywhere. Keep an eye out for them-Switching as much as possible to "GOOD" carbs can make a big impact on your fitness and health effort.

## Recommended Daily Quantities

The Daily Reference Value stipulated by the FDA for people four years or older eating 2000 calories per day is 300 grams of total carbohydrates as shown in the figure below.

| Total Fat | 65 g |
|---|---|
| Saturated Fatty Acids | 20 g |
| Cholesterol | 300 mg |
| Sodium | 2300 mg |
| Potassium | 4700 mg |
| Total Carbohydrate | 300 g |
| Fiber | 25 g |
| Protein | 50 g |

## Proteins

Protein is the second essential nutrient we need to consume on a daily basis. It is the only food source of nitrogen and certain amino acids needed by the body. There are over twenty amino acids and we produce many of them in the body. However, the ones we do not produce, we need to obtain from animal or plant food. Protein is essential for a number of reasons:

- It strengthens our immune system
- It restores daily wear and tear in the body
- It is the substance that hair, skin, and nails are made from
- It supports our growth
- It is the key building block of blood hemoglobin and muscles

The amount of protein we need to consume depends on your body weight, body composition, and fitness goals. The more active we are and the more muscle mass we have, the more protein we should consume.

There are two main external sources of protein:

- Plants
- Animals

Plant protein is found in a wide range of food including beans, nuts, grains, and in some vegetables and fruits. This protein source is considered low quality because its protein lacks some essential amino acids.

**NOTE: In order to obtain all essential amino acids from plant sources, you need to consume a wide variety of them.**

**NOTE: Plant protein can lower cholesterol and is an excellent source of minerals and vitamins.**

Animal protein is found in meat, fish, poultry, eggs, and dairy products. This protein source is considered high-quality protein because its protein contains all the essential amino acids we need.

**NOTE: Most animal protein comes along with high fat that can increase caloric intake and cholesterol. Be cognizant of how much of it you consume.**

Also, be aware that when you consume chicken or any other poultry, the dark meat located on thighs and legs has more fat and thus more calories than the white meat on the breasts. Always consume the leanest protein possible!

**NOTE: Consuming a balanced combination of both the leanest meat and plant proteins may be the best approach to follow.**

Recommended Daily Quantities

The Daily Reference Value stipulated by the FDA for people four years or older eating 2,000 calories per day is 50 grams of protein as shown in the figure below.

| Total Fat | 65 g |
|---|---|
| Saturated Fatty Acids | 20 g |
| Cholesterol | 300 mg |
| Sodium | 2300 mg |
| Potassium | 4700 mg |
| Total Carbohydrate | 300 g |
| Fiber | 25 g |
| Protein | 50 g |

Fats

Fats are the third and final essential nutrient we need to consume on a daily basis. Fats are high in energy and caloric content and thus their consumption should be watched carefully. High-fat food is also prolific in our daily life especially when eating out.

The three types of fats include saturated, polyunsaturated, and monounsaturated.

Saturated Fat is considered BAD because, on top of its high caloric content, when consumed in excess, it can cause arteries to clog. Moreover, when this happens, strokes, heart attacks, and coronary heart disease can result.

Polyunsaturated Fat is considered less harmful than saturated fat. However, it is still highly caloric and its consumption needs to be monitored carefully. On the positive side, omega-3 fat has been found to offer many benefits such as lowering cholesterol levels in the blood and helping with the development of the nervous system and other key body functions.

Monounsaturated Fat is considered the best of the three types. Thus, you should target having a higher intake of this type than the other two whenever possible.

**NOTE: ALL these fats are highly caloric, actually packing close to twice as many calories per unit as protein and carbs.**

Cholesterol

Cholesterol is a necessary substance made by our body. Foods containing animal fat contain varying amounts of cholesterol, which, when added to the level our body makes, can produce harmful excess. This excess can cause clogged arteries that lead to heart-related health issues.

**NOTE: Major dietary sources of cholesterol include cheese, egg yolks, beef, pork, poultry, and shrimp. It is recommended that no more than 300 mg be consumed daily.**

The following figure shows a list of several sources of the poly-unsaturated and monounsaturated fat types.

| Monounsaturated Fat Sources | Omega-6 Polyunsaturated Fat Sources | Omega-3 Polyunsaturated Fat Sources |
|---|---|---|
| Nuts | Soybean oil | Soybean oil |
| Vegetable oils | Corn oil | Canola oil |
| Canola oil | Safflower oil | Walnuts |
| Olive oil | | Flaxseed |
| High oleic safflower oil | | Fish: trout, herring, and |
| Sunflower oil | | salmon |
| Avocado | | |

Recommended Daily Quantities

The Daily Reference Value stipulated by the FDA for people four years or older eating 2000 calories per day is 65 grams of total fat, 20 grams of that amount or less in saturated fat, and 300 milligrams of cholesterol.

Moreover, fats should not make up more that 30 percent of your total daily calorie intake.

**NOTE: Saturated fat should make up 10 percent or less of your consumption if possible!**

| Total Fat | 65 g |
|---|---|
| Saturated Fatty Acids | 20 g |
| Cholesterol | 300 mg |
| Sodium | 2300 mg |
| Potassium | 4700 mg |
| Total Carbohydrate | 300 g |
| Fiber | 25 g |
| Protein | 50 g |

**NOTE: The latest Dietary Guidelines for Americans recommends the following ranges for the proportions of essential nutrients that should be consumed on a daily basis:**

- 45 percent-65 percent of total daily calories from carbohydrates
- 20 percent-35 percent of total daily calories from fats
- 10 percent-35 percent of total daily calories from protein

Vitamins

Vitamins are nutritional organic (of biological origin) substances the body needs to function properly. They should be preferably obtained from food but can be taken orally in pill or tablet form. Following are the thirteen vitamins the body requires to work efficiently:

- Vitamin A
- Vitamin B1
- Vitamin B2
- Vitamin B3
- Vitamin B6
- Vitamin B12
- Folic Acid
- Vitamin C
- Vitamin D
- Vitamin E
- Vitamin K
- Pantothenic Acid
- Biotin

Keep in mind that not getting enough of various vitamins can lead to an assortment of problems. Among these are anemia, blood clotting problems, skin problems, and poor night vision. It is important to ensure that between your food and supplements you are getting these vitamins daily as recommended by health authorities.

**NOTE: ALWAYS consult your doctor or any other credible medical authority before taking any vitamins in any form.**

Minerals

Minerals are nutritional inorganic (of non-biological origin) substances the body also needs to function properly. Like vitamins, they should be preferably obtained from food but can be taken in supplemental form. Following is a list of common minerals our body needs on a daily basis:

- Calcium
- Chlorine
- Chromium
- Copper
- Fluoride
- Iron
- Magnesium
- Manganese
- Molybdenum
- Phosphorus
- Potassium
- Selenium
- Sodium
- Zinc

Here again, keep in mind that not getting enough of these minerals can lead to an assortment of problems. It is important to ensure that between your food and supplements you are getting these minerals daily as recommended by health authorities.

**NOTE: ALWAYS consult your doctor or another credible medical authority before taking any minerals in any form.**

Recommended Daily Quantities:

| Vitamin A | 5000 IU | | Biotin | 300 µg |
|---|---|---|---|---|
| Vitamin C | 60 mg | | Pantothenic acid | 10 mg |
| Calcium | 1000 mg | | Phosphorus | 1000 mg |
| Iron | 18 mg | | Iodine | 150 µg |
| Vitamin D | 400 IU | | Magnesium | 400 mg |
| Vitamin E | 30 IU | | Zinc | 15 mg |
| Vitamin K | 80 µg | | Selenium | 70 µg |
| Thiamin | 1.5 mg | | Copper | 2 mg |
| Riboflavin | 1.7 mg | | Manganese | 2 mg |
| Niacin | 20 mg | | Chromium | 120 µg |
| Vitamin B6 | 2 mg | | Molybdenum | 75 µg |
| Folate | 400 µg | | Chloride | 3400 mg |
| Vitamin B12 | 6 µg | | | |

Fiber

Dietary fiber is the indigestible portion of the plant foods we eat. Fiber is made of soluble and insoluble parts. Soluble fiber is readily fermented in the colon into gas and other active byproducts. Insoluble fiber is the bulk part that absorbs water throughout the digestive system and aids in the defecation process.

Fiber sources are divided according to whether they provide mostly one type or the other. Plant foods contain both types of fiber in varying degrees, depending on certain characteristics.

Soluble fiber can be found in plant foods such as:

- Legumes: peas, soybeans, and other beans
- Oats, rye, and barley
- Fruits and fruit juices: prune juice, plums, berries, bananas, apples, and pears
- Vegetables: broccoli, carrots, and artichokes
- Roots: sweet potatoes and onions

Insoluble fiber can be found in plant foods such as:

- Whole grain food
- Wheat and corn bran
- Nuts and seeds
- Potato and tomato skin
- Flax seed
- Veggies: Green beans, cauliflower, zucchini, and celery
- Fruits: Avocado, and bananas

Recommended Daily Quantities:

| | |
|---|---|
| Total Fat | 65 g |
| Saturated Fatty Acids | 20 g |
| Cholesterol | 300 mg |
| Sodium | 2300 mg |
| Potassium | 4700 mg |
| Total Carbohydrate | 300 g |
| Fiber | 25 g |
| Protein | 50 g |

Water

Water is essential to the body. We cannot survive very long without it! Our body is composed of approximately 60 percent water.

The amount of water you need depends on your weight, height, and level of activity. We get water from a number of the foods we eat, but that is usually not good enough and therefore we need to take additional water to ensure proper hydration.

Key Nutrients Summary

This concludes the overview of the essential nutrients. As you can see, there is a lot of information to absorb and keep in mind in order to help you make informed nutritional choices. However, it is close to impossible and unnecessary to know all of it. We have highlighted he basic principles to remember for making the best choices. We will also repeat them in the planning section later on.

**NOTE: When the foods and drinks you consume lack any of these nutrients, it can have fitness and health implications. Consuming too much of certain nutrients can also have a negative effect. Thus, balanced consumption is the key!**

Food Groups

Another way food is classified is by groups. Following are the food group categories commonly consumed. We present them here because they more closely represent the actual food you consume. You do not ask for carbs at the grocery store or restaurant. We offer you a very brief overview of these groups, what they are made of from a nutrient standpoint, and their energy balance impact.

I - Fats, Oils & Sweets

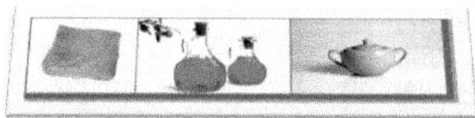

This category represents the HIGHEST caloric content foods. We recommend you consume these sporadically or never at all. That is because, as you learned earlier, fats contain almost twice as many calories per unit of measure than the other two primary nutrients: carbohydrates and protein. Moreover, saturated fats are not very good for you, as you learned.

| Energy Source | Calories per gram |
|---|---|
| Fats | 9 |
| Proteins | 4 |
| Carbohydrates | 4 |

**NOTE: Processed sugars, found in most sweets such as regular soda products, candies, and a number of other "sweet" products with high sugar content, are also very high in caloric content.**

II - Meat, Fish, Eggs, Beans & Peas

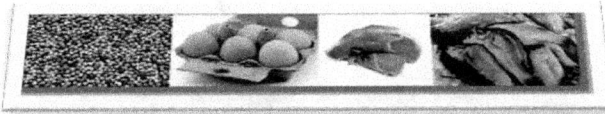

This category includes the next layer of food with high caloric content. Meat, fish, and eggs have varying degrees of and types of fats in addition to their high protein content. In addition to high protein content, beans and peas have high natural sugar content, which raises their caloric content enough to make this category.

III - Milk, Cheese & Yogurt

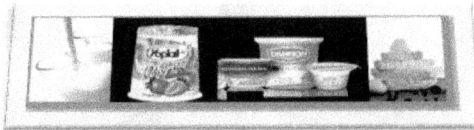

This category includes foods that have the next layer of caloric content because of high fat content. However, they also contain high amounts of the important mineral, calcium. Thus, the USDA (US Department of Agriculture) recommends intake of the low fat versions of these foods.

IV - Bread, Cereals, Rice, Pasta & Potatoes

This category includes foods with generally lower caloric content than those above. Breads, cereals, and pasta made using multigrains have been found to be much better than those made using processed flour. Sweet varieties of potatoes are better than white varieties. The USDA highly recommends consuming foods in this category.

V - Fruits & Veggies

This category is the lowest caloric content category of foods. In addition, they provide a broad variety and quantity of essential vitamins and minerals. Thus, the USDA recommends high frequency and volume consumption of all of them.

VI - Water

Water has no actual nutritional value per se or any caloric content. Nevertheless, it is highly critical for human survival.

**NOTE: Water is valuable in efforts to improve and maintain good fitness and health.**

Foods' Nutrient Levels

The figure on the following page provides a quick summary of food groups and their relative generic energy and nutritional content. We provide it to allow you quick access to key nutritional characteristics of several general food categories.

Go to www.fitnessprotcols.com/book/forms.pdf if you want to download a larger full color version of this diagram.

## Nutrient & Energy Content Levels

**Legend:**
- High or Bad Range
- Med. or Ok Range
- Low or Good Range
- None or Very Low

| Foods Category | Carbs | Fats | Protein | Vitamins | Minerals | Calories |
|---|---|---|---|---|---|---|
| Fruits | L | | | | | L |
| Vegies | L | | | | | L |
| Grains | M | | | | | L |
| Beans | | | | | | L |
| Eggs | | | | M | | L |
| Poultry | | M | | | | M |
| Fish | | M | | | M | M |
| Nuts | | H | L | | L | H |
| Dairy | L | H | L | | L | H |
| Meat | | H | | | | H |
| Sugar | H | | | | | H |
| Oils | | H | | L | L | H |

Food appears on the left side and the nutritional aspects appear across the top row. The rectangles found at the intersection of the food and nutritional factor give you a generic sense of the level of the factor in that food category. Note that because foods that have high fat content will also have high caloric content, they appear with the (H) high rectangles.

This concludes the Nutritional and Energy Balance Sections.

Activity Balance

Activity Balance is the dynamic involving expenditure of the right amount of time working on exercises that stimulate and strengthen the body's key fitness-related systems to the extent required by your fitness needs. The cardiovascular, skeletal, and muscular systems need to be exercised at regular intervals with varying degrees of intensity and duration in order to achieve the optimal level of fitness that meets your need or want. The figure below shows a model of the key elements involved in the Activity Dynamic.

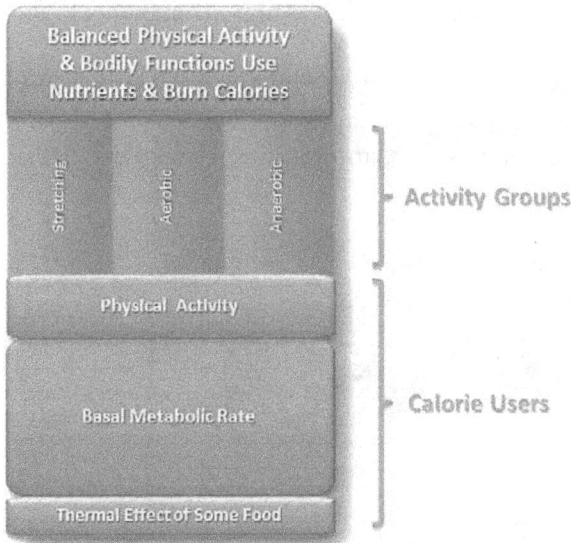

Since people have different fitness level needs depending on what they must do or like to do, the goal is to develop a fitness level appropriate to their specific wants or needs. That means the amount, frequency, and level of physical activity will vary accordingly. Moreover, since everyone starts at a different level, the time to accomplish the desired fitness level will also be different.

The best approach to improving fitness is a planned and careful approach. You will need to consider your current condition, past history, skill level, and other factors.

**NOTE: ALWAYS consult your doctor or other credible medical authority before taking on physical activity.**

How the Body Works

The reasons we want to become and remain fit are straightforward. Improved fitness should lead to increased physical and mental energy, additional muscular strength, improved physical flexibility, more cardiovascular endurance, and enhanced physical agility, coordination, and balance. All these, in turn, should enable us to live a more productive and joyful life. Overall, better fitness should make us look and feel much better!

Improving your physical fitness will involve work with the skeletal, muscular, cardiovascular, and respiratory systems. Let us go over each of them briefly.

I - The Skeletal System

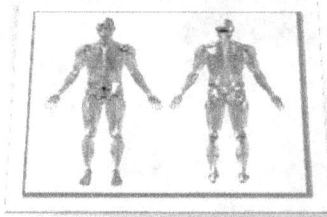

This system includes all the bones, joints, and ligaments in the body. This system holds us together and enables us to move, walk, run, lift, push, etc. Our bones are made of living tissue. Bone mass is maintained by a balance between the activity of the osteoblasts cells that form bone and the osteoclasts cells that break it down. Osteoblasts are constantly bringing calcium into bones to make them stronger and osteoclasts use up calcium from bones. Physical activity increases the rate at which osteoblasts strengthen bones. On the other hand, inactivity slows osteoblastic activity thus weakening bones. This means activities placing force on bones should strengthen them.

II - The Muscular System

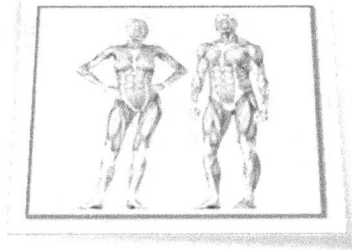

This system includes all the muscles and tendons in the body. This system covers the skeleton and enables it to stay together and enable our movement. Muscles are the key to fitness. They grow and become stronger with use. Moreover, the more muscle mass we build, the more efficient we become at burning calories. That is because muscles use a lot more energy than any other tissue in our body.

Activities focused on the larger muscles groups located in our legs and buttocks will yield the most benefit concerning your basal (at rest) metabolic rate. However, a balanced approach is always best; thus, strength training of all muscle groups will yield the most benefit. Focus on particular muscle groups based on your particular situation because we all have different fitness needs.

III - The Cardiovascular System

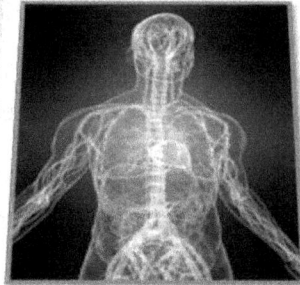

This system includes the heart, arteries, and blood vessels. This system enables blood circulation with delivery of oxygen obtained from the air we breathe into our lungs. Moreover, it delivers nutrients from digested food to the body systems that need it. The heart is a muscle and, like other muscles, the more we use it, the stronger it gets. When we are very active, muscle uses a lot of oxygen to keep up. The heart thus needs to work harder and over time gets stronger. This results in better cardiovascular capacity, which allows you to do more activity with less effort. Moreover, once at rest the heart actually works less. Top athletes and other fit people are known to have very low heart rates when at rest.

IV - The Respiratory System

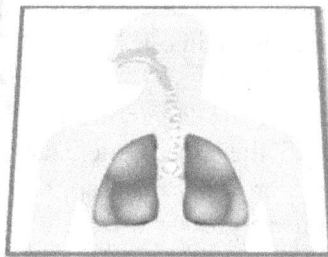

This system includes the lungs and the air passages such as the nose that deliver air we breathe to the lungs. Some consider this part of the cardiovascular system. The system delivers oxygen into the blood when we inhale and carbon dioxide out of the blood and out of our body when we exhale. Breathing is a critical aspect of fitness and closely related, if not a part of, the cardiovascular process.

Now let us look at how it all works together in the context of your fitness.

Physical Activity and Exercise

There are two basic types of physical activity or exercise:

- Aerobic
- Anaerobic

Aerobic activity, also known as cardio, is the type that makes you breathe hard. It is good for the heart because it makes it beat fast in order to pump blood around the body to deliver oxygen to the muscles being used. Aerobic exercises include walking, running, swimming, dancing, biking, rowing, etc. The more active you become, the more efficient your body will also become at pumping oxygen to your muscles.

Running

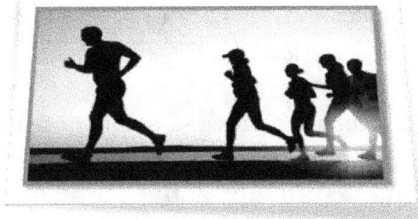

Anaerobic activity, also known as strength training, does not make your heart beat faster. This is activity good for the muscle because when you use muscles they grow and get stronger. This type involves short but intense activity. Anaerobic exercise involves a variety of weight lifting and muscle building activities. A typical workout involves multiple sets of routines focused on particular muscles or muscle groups.

Weights

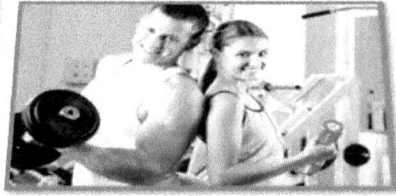

Why Physical Activity is GOOD for YOU

The Advisory Committee on the Dietary Guidelines for Americans 2010 reports uncovering strong and consistent evidence indicating that physically active people are at reduced risk of becoming overweight or obese. Moreover, they uncovered strong evidence showing that even overweight or obese who are physically active experience health benefits similar to people in much better shape.

Additionally, the committee found strong and consistent evidence indicating that compared to those less active, physically active people:

- Have higher levels of health-related fitness.
- Run a lower risk of developing many chronic or disabling conditions.
- Experience lower rates of a number of chronic diseases.

**NOTE: Being habitually active appears to benefit people regardless of age, sex, race/ethnicity, or socioeconomic status. People with physical or cognitive disabilities, such as ADDH, benefit from activity.**

They found further consistent evidence that shows that physical activity provides benefit for weight stability.

Preparation

## How Much and How Often is Better

Accordingly, they recommend 60 minutes or more of physical activity for children and adolescents. Moreover, 150 to 300 minutes per week of moderate-intensity physical activity, or 75 to 150 minutes per week of vigorous-intensity physical activity for adults and older adults. An equivalent combination of the two is recommended to help maintain body weight over time.

**NOTE: Many experts recommend at least ten thousand steps be ideally completed every day. These steps should include normal walking activity and planned physical activity. A portion of the planned activity should be strenuous enough to get your heart rate up to target for at least ten or fifteen minutes.**

### Activity and Weigh Loss

The Advisory Committee found additional strong evidence that a large dose of physical activity is needed for weight loss greater than 5 percent of body weight. Adults found to have been most successful at achieving weight loss combined calorie restriction with increased physical activity.

Adding credence to our suggested balanced approach to fitness, strong evidence also showed that adults who participated in physical activity during weight loss improved body composition more so than those who lost weight by reducing calories alone. The end benefit of using both approaches was muscle mass preservation and belly fat/waist size reduction.

### Stretching

Another highly beneficial type of activity or exercise is stretching. There are many ways to stretch. More recently, Yoga practices have become one of, if not the most popular, form of this activity type. Stretching is a form of anaerobic exercise, as it helps with muscle strengthening. Besides being highly recommended prior to aerobic and anaerobic workout stretching, it is also excellent to help make you more flexible. Yoga practitioners are amazingly flexible.

Being flexible offers some tremendous day-to-day advantages, as you do even some of the most basic things in life. Flexibility also helps prevent sometimes-painful injuries resulting from other activities such as pulled muscles and tendons, etc.

Samples of Stretching Poses

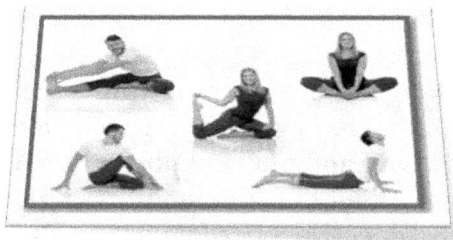

Warming up and Cooling Down

Another essential factor is warming up. Warming up and stretching before exercising reduces the chance of injury. A warm-up should raise your heart rate, and you should do it for at least five minutes. Riding a stationary bike (with low resistance) is a good warm-up, but there are plenty of other ways. Likewise, after strenuous exercise you should cool down and stretch. Walking (at normal speed) and riding a stationary bike (with low resistance) are both good ways to cool down.

Technological Fitness Aids

Significant progress on technology gadgets aids in monitoring and tracking physical activity. Pedometers and heart rate monitors are prolific and relatively inexpensive. More recently, apps for smartphones supporting many aspects of fitness have become available. Monitoring and tracking certain aspects such as weight and daily steps have been linked with successful fitness outcomes and fitness maintenance.

This concludes the section on how the body works. Following is a summary with the key takeaways from the section.

## Key Takeaways

1. Energy balance is MOST critical

When we consume more calories than we burn on a daily basis, we gain weight! **You need to be VIGILANT about the intake of calories.** Keep in mind that around 20 percent of the food you take in will most likely contain around 80 percent of the calories overall. Concentrate on that 20 percent to manage you caloric intake. Look for fats as high-leverage items, as they are the primary calorie culprits. Leverage means that a small adjustment in fat intake can make a big difference in caloric intake downward. **To help you monitor proper energy balance, you should get on a scale daily to watch your weight.** This is very important to help you achieve and maintain good balance. Doing so is a MUST!

2. Watch your fat intake

Fats are high in calories and while some, such as omega-3 fatty acids, are good for you, they still pack high calories. On the other hand, saturated fats are not only high in calories but too much of them can eventually kill you!

The Advisory Committee on the Dietary Guidelines for Americans 2010 reports finding strong evidence indicating that **excessive intake of saturated fat is highly related to increased risk of cardiovascular disease, and type 2 diabetes (T2D). Moreover, decreasing saturated fat intake showed improved lowering of the bad cholesterol causing CVD and decreased insulin resistance that causes T2D.**

Remember that fat has twice the caloric content of protein and carbs. **Watch for those fat calories and AVOID saturated ones at all cost.**

3. Watch your simple sugar carbs intake

Simple sugars are high in calories and the digested and unused portion gets stored away as fat in your body.

141

**Avoid simple sugar foods such as table sugar, sugar-sweetened soft drinks, white potatoes, and white rice at all cost.**

4.  Eat smaller-portion balanced meals more often

Try to consume five or six meals containing balanced nutrients throughout your day. Make sure all meals have a similar quantity of good fat, lean protein, and good carbs.

5.  Consume balanced minimum recommended daily amounts

The Advisory Committee on the Dietary Guidelines for Americans 2010 also reported finding no optimal proportion of protein, fat, and carbs that enhances weight loss or maintenance. Their analysis of the available research concluded that ultimately decreasing caloric intake is what best leads to weight loss and increases the likelihood of weight maintenance.

Nutritional approaches that reduce caloric intake and stick to currently recommended proportions of 10-35 percent protein, 45-65 percent carbohydrate, and 20-35 percent fat are most appropriate to help you become more fit and to remain so.

Approaches that promote intakes of less than 45 percent carbohydrate or more than 35 percent protein were found difficult to adhere to and were not any more effective than caloric control approaches. Moreover, low carb and high protein approaches can present health risks, and are not recommended.

**Ensure your meals contain the daily minimum recommended amounts of fat, protein, and carbohydrates. Vitamins and minerals are also recommended.**

6.  Avoid eating out at all cost

Eating out, while convenient, makes it hard to find food that meets the above-mentioned criteria. Portions are larger and the ingredients are intended to entice you to come back for more.

**There is excess sugar, sodium, and fat galore out there!** It will make your fitness effort very challenging!

7.   Drink enough water

Water is not only necessary (critical), but it is great for weight management and maintenance. It keeps you hydrated and cleansed inside. If your urine is not somewhat clear when you go to the bathroom, you may not be drinking enough for your needs.

8.   Building muscle mass is key to fitness

Muscles are efficient at burning energy; thus, the more mass you have the better you will burn calories while at rest. Strength training should be an important element of your fitness approach.

9.   Easy does it

You do not need to run long distances or fast to start with. Start easy and slow and your body will lead you to the next levels. The key is consistently moving and ensuring you heart rate gets elevated for a portion of the time you work out as long as you have medical consent for your activity. The ultimate and ideal target is ten thousand steps a day or more depending on your goal or needs. You can accomplish this in about an hour depending on how fast you walk or run. ALWAYS stretch before starting any type of physical activity!

10. Form Habits

If you are consistent, you will form habits much faster. When that happens, it should make any new activity feel like part of your normal life. In fact, as time passes you will need to do these things. Eventually, you will feel better and better after doing activities and that will reinforce the activity.

Now that you have completed the basic section, you are ready to move to the next section intended to establish your baseline or starting point.

## Establish Your Baseline

This part will help you establish your fitness baseline.

About Baselines

Baselining is a highly useful exercise because it sets the basis for understanding where you are and for the reasons why you are where you are. This information is useful to help you better understand your situation and develop goals and plans that are more likely to lead to success. As the figure below illustrates, this is the second of four steps intended to get you ready for a new and more effective fitness approach for you.

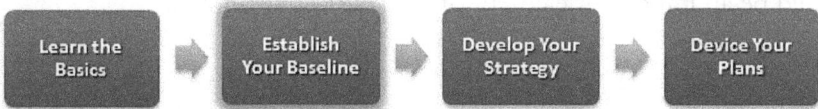

Here you will identify you current health and fitness conditions, consider possible root causes, and choose your priorities.

You current condition aspects include basic health and fitness facts such as heart rate, blood pressure, weight, BMI, waist diameter, etc.

Root causes are the reasons why such conditions may exist. Sometimes these may seem obvious but when you dig a little deeper, you may find the true underlying reason(s). In addition, when you do, the solution to the problem can be much more effective. This is what we call working on the right problem.

# Step 1 - Your Current Conditions

This step will help document your current condition.

Baselining

A baseline is a point of reference or the starting point. The baseline is useful to help set realistic goals and enable the monitoring of progress toward goal achievement.

The Baselining Process

The baselining process involves collecting information in the following four categories:

1. Key Fitness Metrics
2. Key Fitness Capabilities
3. Daily Energy Balance Patterns
4. Daily Lifestyle Activity Pattern

The information collected will provide great insight you will use for goal setting and strategy development.

Establish Your Baseline

1 - Key Fitness Metrics

The key fitness metrics we want to baseline include:

- Waist Size
- Body Weight
- BMI, or Body Mass Index
- RMR, or Resting Metabolic Rate
- RHR, or Resting Heart Rate
- BP, or Blood Pressure

Waist Size is a measurement of the diameter of your waist near the belly button.

Body Weight is a measurement of your body weight taken first thing in the morning on an empty stomach and preferably with nothing on.

BMI, or body mass index, is a calculation of body fat based on height and weight that applies to adult men and women. BMI is a much more accurate fitness metric than weight.

RMR, or resting metabolic rate, is a calculation representing the estimated minimum amount of energy in calories required to keep your body functioning, including your heart beating, lungs breathing, and body temperature for a period of twenty-four hours.

RHR, or resting heart rate, is a measurement of the number of heartbeats per minute at which your heart pumps blood while you are at rest.

The best time to measure is in the morning, after a good night's sleep, and just before you get out of bed. The two best ways to take it are either on your wrist (radial pulse) or on your neck (carotid pulse).

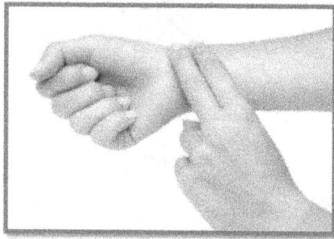

To take it on your wrist, simply put your index finger and third finger tips on the thumb side of either wrist as shown in this figure. Hold the fingertips gently until you feel the beats. Count the number of pulses in ten seconds and multiply that number by six to obtain the actual reading.

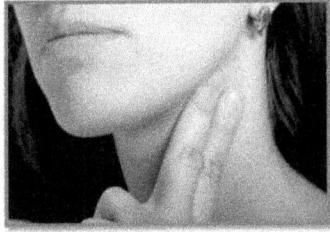

To take it on your neck, simply put your index finger and third fingertips right below your jaw along the windpipe and throat as shown in this figure. Hold the fingertips gently until you feel the beats. Count the number of pulses in ten seconds and multiply that number by six to obtain the actual reading.

BP, or blood pressure, is a measurement of the pressure exerted by circulating blood upon blood vessels' walls. Blood pressure measurements involve two numbers, the systolic pressure and diastolic pressure.

Systolic stands for the highest pressure and diastolic for the lowest in the circulatory system's blood vessels. You can take your BP measurement with a special medical instrument on the inside of the elbow on the upper arm portion right by the brachial artery as shown in the figure below.

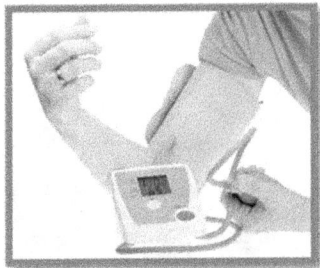

You can also take BP measurement on the wrist with a different type of instrument as shown on the figure below.

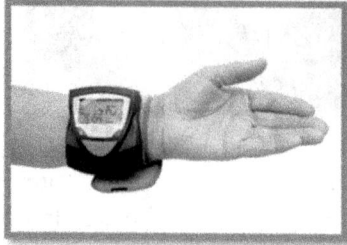

Additional Information

In order to calculate your BMI and RMR, you will need to enter your gender, age, weight, and height into the following form. Before starting to enter data, you need to take your pulse using the procedure above. You need to take your blood pressure also. If you do not have a blood pressure machine at home, you can locate a free one to use in most pharmacies.

Key Fitness Metric Baseline

Once you have obtained all the measurements, you can capture them using the following form.

| Gender | F | M |
|---|---|---|
| Age | | |
| Height in Inches | | |
| Weight in Pounds | | |
| Waist in Inches | | |
| At Rest Heart Rete | | |
| Systolic Blood Pressure | | |
| Diastolic Blood Pressure | | |

2 - Key Fitness Capabilities

Next, we want to document your current fitness capabilities. We want to baseline six fitness capabilities:

- Flexibility
- Endurance
- Agility
- Strength
- Coordination
- Energy

We have chosen a simple approach to baseline these capabilities. However, approaches that are more formal are available. Feel free to take the time to find them on the Web and use them to give you a more formal assessment if you so desire. Ultimately, the idea here is for you to improve those capabilities you deem most important given your needs and wants.

Let us take a quick look at a basic definition and illustration for each of them before you proceed with the baselining process.

Physical Flexibility is the ability to move our joints or muscles through their full range of motion.

Cardiovascular Endurance, or aerobic capacity, is the ability of our cardiovascular system to deliver oxygen to our body, and of our muscles and tissues to utilize the delivered oxygen, thus preventing fatigue.

Agility is the ability to move our body quickly and accurately without losing our balance.

Physical or muscular strength is our ability to lift, hold, pull, or push physical objects with our arms and or legs.

Coordination is the ability to integrate the aforementioned capabilities in order to accomplish the most effective body movements possible.

Energy gives us the ability to sustain physical and/or mental efforts for prolonged periods.

Fitness Capabilities Baseline

Take a minute to think about each of the above capabilities and use the following form to assess your current level. Enter any number between one and five. One means your capability is low and five means high.

| Flexibility | |
| Endurance | |
| Agility | |
| Strength | |
| Coordination | |
| Energy | |

3 - Daily Energy Balance Patterns

As you recall from the Energy Balance section, the most successful fitness improvement efforts result from a good combination of caloric intake reduction and an increase in caloric utilization.

In this part of the baseline process, we will document your typical daily and weekly eating and activity patterns. The idea is to get a general sense of what and how much you eat, and of when and where you eat. We are looking to identify areas where a small or easy adjustment can cause a big impact. We are also looking to determine your level of consistency in what, when, where, and how you eat and what you do.

**NOTE: Consistency is a key success factor of fitness improvement.**

Eating and activity patterns are mostly habitual. That means that much of what we do happens outside our awareness. Therefore, the process of documenting our patterns and uncovering certain aspects of them can be extremely helpful. People who complete this are typically amazed at some of the things they uncover. It can give you great insight! It should be time well spent!

Eating Patterns

The ideal outcome of this exercise will be to be able to identify 20 percent of the food and drinks that provide 80 percent of your daily caloric intake. The top suspects will be items you consume containing high fat and/or simple (bad) carbohydrates. All fats are high in calories and simple carbohydrates turn to sugar fast. Any excess sugar in the blood will eventually end up stored as fat once the liver and muscles get what they need. That is the target zone!

Use the form on the following page to document your current eating and drinking patterns. Ideally, unless you are very consistent, you should attempt to capture your daily eating pattern for each day of a full week. It would be most useful if you can complete it in real time. There is no need to get a super accurate number. Try to figure out the nutrients and calories to the best of your ability. There is a lot of information about it on the Web.

If you prefer a larger copy, you may download it from www.fitnessprotocols.com/book/forms.pdf.

## Daily Food Intake Pattern

| | Breakfast | Morning Snack | Lunch | Afternoon Snack | Dinner | Evening Snack 1 | Evening Snack 2 |
|---|---|---|---|---|---|---|---|
| Monday | | | | | | | |
| Tuesday | | | | | | | |
| Wednesday | | | | | | | |
| Thursday | | | | | | | |
| Friday | | | | | | | |
| Saturday | | | | | | | |
| Sunday | | | | | | | |

Food Categories: Cups of Veggies, Cups of Fruit, Tbs. of Oil, Eq. Oz. of Protein, Eq. Oz. of Grains, Glasses of Water

Food Amount

Meal Details: Meal Time, Meal Location, Meal Cost, Meal Duration, Meal Mood

Meal Data

Preparation

Activity Patterns

Capturing your activity pattern will also provide great information that will give you useful insight into how you spend some of your time related to all activities you are involved in.

Use the form on the following page to document your current activity pattern. Ideally, unless you are very consistent, you should attempt to capture your daily pattern for each day of the week. It would be most useful if you can complete it on a daily basis.

If you prefer a larger copy, you may download it from www.fitnessprotocols.com/book/forms.pdf.

| Regular | Cardio | Strength | Flexibility |
|---------|--------|----------|-------------|

## Daily Physical Activity Pattern

| Day of Week | Mon | Tue | Web | Thu | Fri | Sat | Sun |
|-------------|-----|-----|-----|-----|-----|-----|-----|
| Distance Covered | | | | | | | |
| Number of Steps | | | | | | | |
| Number of Reps | | | | | | | |
| Number of Sets | | | | | | | |
| Activity Intensity | | | | | | | |
| Activity Duration | | | | | | | |
| Time of Day | | | | | | | |
| Activity Location | | | | | | | |

4 - Daily Lifestyle Activity Pattern

Your daily lifestyle activity pattern is the final set of information you need to collect. This is an important set of data! It will show how you distribute your time among three key categories of time:

- Resting
- Working
- Living

Use the form on the following page to document your time over the next week. At least once a day record your time.

If you prefer a larger copy, you may download it from www.fitnessprotocols.com/book/forms.pdf.

| | Monday | Tuesday | Wednesday | Thursday | Friday | Saturday | Sunday |
|---|---|---|---|---|---|---|---|

## Daily Lifestyle Activity Pattern

| Activity | Type | Activity Time | Total Time |
|---|---|---|---|
| Resting | Laying down | | |
| | Sleeping | | |
| Working | Moving | | |
| | Sitting | | |
| Living | Moving | | |
| | Sitting | | |

Additional Fitness Metrics

If you have not done so recently, it would be very useful to get a complete physical examination done. These physicals include a battery of tests and blood work that provide ideal baseline information beyond what we are capturing here.

Some important data from the test results would include:

- Total Cholesterol:_____
- HDL Cholesterol:_____
- LDL Cholesterol:_____
- Blood Sugar:_____

It would be good to have this information at the onset to both give you an idea for another layer of your condition and to show you later how your fitness improvement affects these critical indicators and predictors of fitness and health.

Congratulations on completing this section! We will use the information gathered later in another section.

## Step 2 - Finding the Root Reasons

This step will help you identify the root reason(s) for your current fitness condition.

Possible Reasons

Your current fitness condition results from a number of causes. In this section, we will help you explore possible reasons. This is an important effort because it will pinpoint the areas and aspects that you should consider when you devise your new fitness approach to achieve you goal.

Many fitness programs will have you "jump" into diets and exercise plans without first helping you explore the reasons behind your current fitness condition. This may be one reason why a very low percent of those people are able to remain fit after improvement efforts.

In order to maintain your fitness improvement, once you achieve it, you should identify, understand, and resolve the underlying reasons for your condition. Otherwise, the same reasons that got you in your current situation may still be there and can get you right back where you started in short order.

Digging for the Roots

Outside of any medical issues or genetic influences, your fitness condition is most likely the result of one or both of the following:

- You have not been eating right.
- You have not been active enough.

However, the search for reasons will most likely not end at this first level. There are usually multiple layers of reasons. Hence, you should keep asking why until you get to the bottom ones. Let us examine additional layers next.

Preparation

The Next Layers

If your fitness is not what it should be because you have not been eating right, one or more of the following reasons maybe behind that:

- Better food has not been readily available to you.
- Eating better has not been very convenient for you.
- You have been eating out of habit or tradition.
- Eating better has not been that important to you.
- You have lacked knowledge about better nutrition.
- You have been eating food you like to eat and/or enjoy eating.
- You have not been able to afford better food.
- You have not had the time to eat better.
- Other

On the other hand, if your fitness is not what it should be because you have not been as active as you should, one or more of the following reasons maybe behind that:

- Being active has not been convenient for you.
- Your activity level has been a matter of habit.
- Being more active has not been that important to you.
- You have not been aware of or known much about physical activity.
- You have not been able to afford being more active.
- A physical or health condition has prevented or limited your activity.
- You have not had enough time to be more active.
- You highly dislike doing physical activity.
- Other

So far, we have identified two of the most likely top reasons, each with their own list of potential reasons. However, you may not be done yet and you may need to dig further. Next, you should examine the ones you choose to see and what might be behind each of them. The process should continue until you get to the ultimate root cause.

**NOTE: Just like the weeds in the yard will keep coming back until you take all their roots out, your fitness struggle will not end until you identify and resolve its entire root causes.**

Let us look at an example at the next level. Assuming one of the key reasons for not being more active has been your lack of time, you should try to figure out why that is so. You need to try to understand the reason behind your time constraint. Otherwise, left unresolved, time can continue to be a limitation or an impediment to your being more active. Interestingly, time happens to be one of the top mentioned reasons for people's low levels of activity in the USA. Work, school, and family matters top the list of reasons why time is a constraint to being more active. Let us try to find the underlying causes of your situation.

Identifying Your Top Reason(s)

Now that you have a better idea of how this works, take some time to identify and rank your top reasons. Once you have them, we will help you identify what may be behind them. Use the forms on the following page to start reviewing our proposed list, adding to it if necessary and then ranking your top three reasons.

To rank them simply enter a "1" for your top reason, a "2" for the next, and a "3" for the third. It is fine if you have only one or two. You may also enter you own reasons, if those listed did not cover it for you. If that is the case, use the blank spaces to enter another reason, and then choose your top three reasons from the list. Once you do one form, touch the next one if it applies to you.

If you prefer a larger copy, you may download it from www.fitnessprotocols.com/book/forms.pdf.

# Preparation

## You have not been more active because…

| | Possible Reasons | My Rank |
|---|---|---|
| **I have not been more active because…** | Being active has not been convenient for me | |
| | My activity level has been a matter of habit | |
| | Being more active has not been that important to me | |
| | I had not been aware of and/or knew much about physical activity | |
| | I have not been able to afford being more active | |
| | A physical or health condition has prevented or limited my activity | |
| | I have not had enough time to be more active | |
| | I highly dislike doing physical activity | |
| | Enter other | |
| | Enter other | |

## You may not have been eating right because…

| | Possible Reasons | My Rank |
|---|---|---|
| **I have not been eating Right because…** | Better food has not been easily available to me | |
| | Eating better has not been very convenient for me | |
| | I have been eating out of habit or tradition | |
| | Eating better has not been that important to me | |
| | I have not had any or enough knowledge about better nutrition | |
| | I have been eating food I like to eat and/or enjoy eating | |
| | I have not been able to afford better food | |
| | I have not had the time to eat better | |
| | Enter other | |
| | Enter other | |

The Next Layer

Now that you have your top three chosen reasons behind each, you need to explore each of the top three, at least one more level down, to try to identify the underlying cause. These causes will be very useful in the next section where you will devise your new approach to fitness improvement and maintenance.

As you read before, the most effective fitness approaches should include both nutrition and activity elements. Aside from any medical reasons that prevent or limit your physical activity, you should do all that is possible to find solutions to all your top reasons.

Use the forms on the following pages to help you identify the root for each of areas respectively.

If you prefer larger copies, you may download them from www.fitnessprotocols.com/book/forms.pdf.

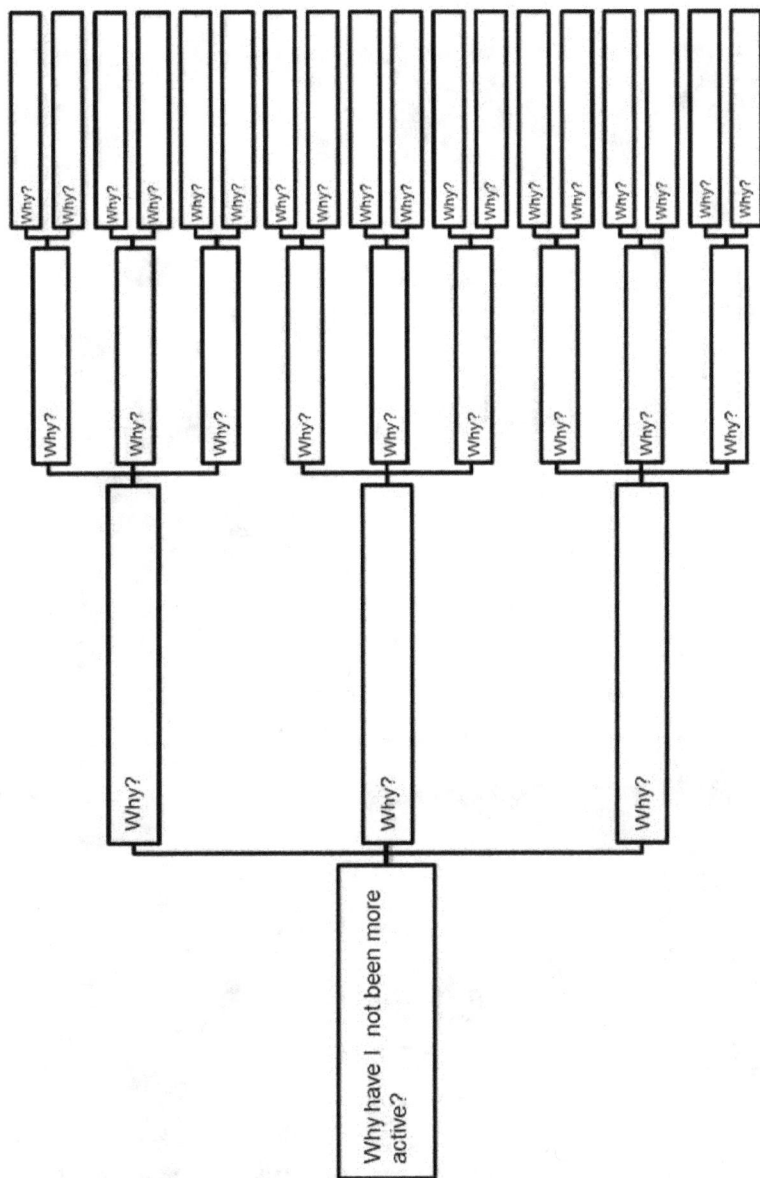

Why have I not been more active?

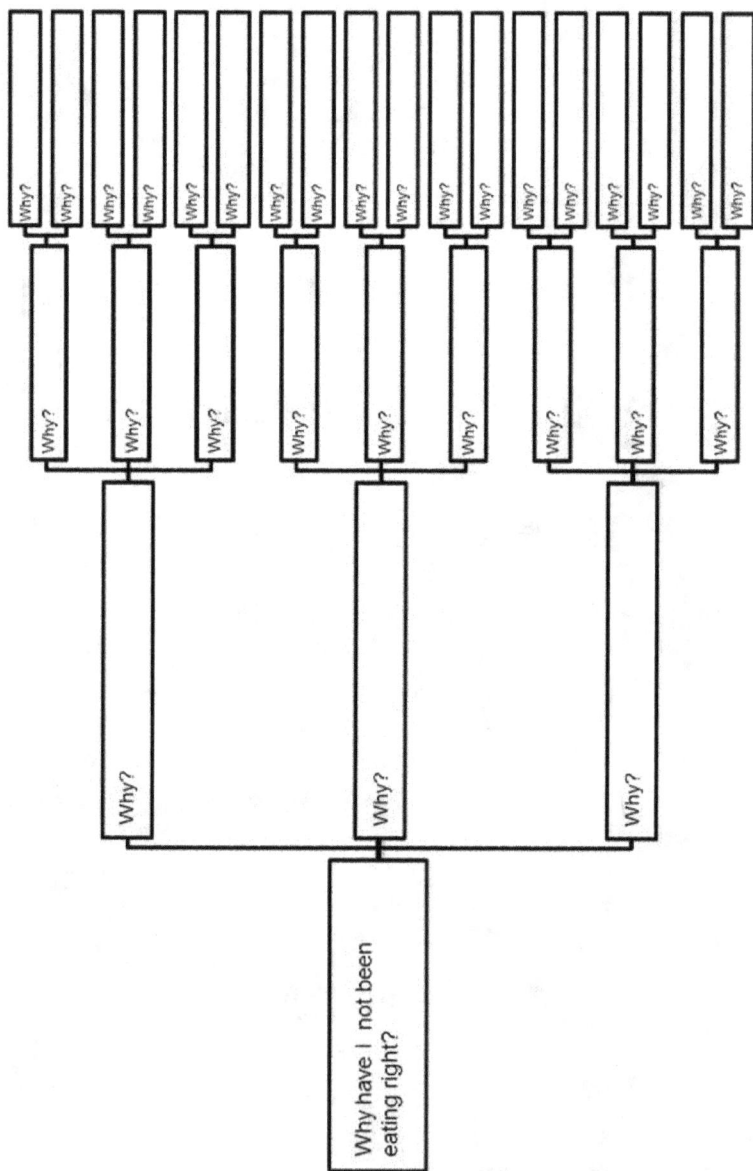

## Develop Your Strategy

This part will help you set your improvement targets and develop a strategy to help you accomplish them.

About Your Strategy

This is the third phase of the preparation process as you can see in the figure below. Here we will help you accomplish two things: first, we will enable you to set your improvement targets, and then devise strategies to help you strengthen and maintain the improvement.

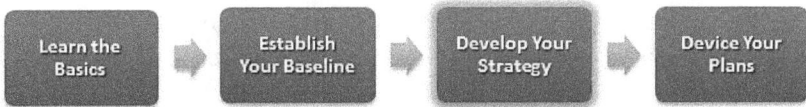

Strategies are behind most successful endeavors. They seem to be imperative for success! Having a strategy also should help build your confidence because it will provide direction and guidance for your efforts. Therefore, your time and effort to develop it should be well worth the effort!

Improvement Targets

The first step is to set your targets. The targets will be set according to your baseline results, your needs and wants, and the available fitness and health guidelines set forth by medical experts. The set targets will determine the strategies and tactics you will need to apply in order to achieve the targets.

The Strategy

The second step is to develop your strategy. As we pointed out earlier in the "Learn the Basics" section, research has consistently shown that the most effective approach to fitness improvement involves both nutrition and activity efforts. The framework for your strategy is straightforward, involving only four categories, as illustrated by the figure that follows on the next page.

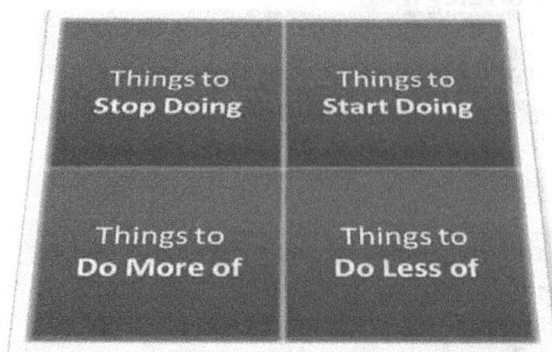

Each category will include a set of recommended actions intended to help achieve respective objectives and specific targets.

In most cases, the strategy will involve a set of recommendations to stop and start, do more of, or do less of, the things that can enable the reduction of caloric intake and the increase of physical activity. Moreover, the strategy will provide you with direction and guidance to help you resolve some of the key reasons that put you in your current condition.

## Step 1 - Set Your Key Targets

This step will help you set your improvement targets.

About Key Fitness Targets

Targets are the fixed goals or objectives, which you are aiming at. The Key Fitness Targets include the most important fitness parameters, which directly or indirectly indicate your fitness level. These include BMI, weight, waist size, RHR, and energy balance. Health and fitness experts have determined the recommended target level values. However, in some cases, you may wish to aim for a lower or higher level depending on your condition, circumstances, needs, or wants. You may choose whatever level you desire.

Your BMI and Weight Targets

The table on the following page shows BMI levels according to height and weight on the bottom row. Since weight is the only controllable parameter in the BMI calculation, the target parameter is your weight. Start by putting a circle on your height. Then follow along the same row until you find the number closest to your current weight and circle that. From that point move all the way down to the bottom row to identify your current BMI value. In order to get to what your target weight should be, follow along the BMI row until you get to 24. Then move up that column back up to the row corresponding to your height. The number at that intersection should be your target weight.

If you prefer a larger copy, you may download it from www.fitnessprotocols.com/book/forms.pdf.

| Height | NORMAL RANGE | | | | | | OVERWEIGHT RANGE | | | | | OBESE RANGE | | | | | | | | | |
|---|---|---|---|---|---|---|---|---|---|---|---|---|---|---|---|---|---|---|---|---|---|
| 58 | 91 | 96 | 100 | 105 | 110 | 115 | 119 | 124 | 129 | 134 | 138 | 143 | 148 | 153 | 158 | 162 | 167 | 172 | 177 | 181 | 186 |
| 59 | 94 | 99 | 104 | 109 | 114 | 119 | 124 | 128 | 133 | 138 | 143 | 148 | 153 | 158 | 163 | 168 | 173 | 178 | 183 | 188 | 193 |
| 60 | 97 | 102 | 107 | 112 | 118 | 123 | 128 | 133 | 138 | 143 | 148 | 153 | 158 | 163 | 168 | 174 | 179 | 184 | 189 | 194 | 199 |
| 61 | 100 | 106 | 111 | 116 | 122 | 127 | 132 | 137 | 143 | 148 | 153 | 158 | 164 | 169 | 174 | 180 | 185 | 190 | 195 | 201 | 206 |
| 62 | 104 | 109 | 115 | 120 | 126 | 131 | 136 | 142 | 147 | 153 | 158 | 164 | 169 | 175 | 180 | 186 | 191 | 196 | 202 | 207 | 213 |
| 63 | 107 | 113 | 118 | 124 | 130 | 135 | 141 | 146 | 152 | 158 | 163 | 169 | 175 | 180 | 186 | 191 | 197 | 203 | 208 | 214 | 220 |
| 64 | 110 | 116 | 122 | 128 | 134 | 140 | 145 | 151 | 157 | 163 | 169 | 174 | 180 | 186 | 192 | 197 | 204 | 209 | 215 | 221 | 227 |
| 65 | 114 | 120 | 126 | 132 | 138 | 144 | 150 | 156 | 162 | 168 | 174 | 180 | 186 | 192 | 198 | 204 | 210 | 216 | 222 | 228 | 234 |
| 66 | 118 | 124 | 130 | 136 | 142 | 148 | 155 | 161 | 167 | 173 | 179 | 186 | 192 | 198 | 204 | 210 | 216 | 223 | 229 | 235 | 241 |
| 67 | 121 | 127 | 134 | 140 | 146 | 153 | 159 | 166 | 172 | 178 | 185 | 191 | 198 | 204 | 211 | 217 | 223 | 230 | 236 | 242 | 249 |
| 68 | 125 | 131 | 138 | 144 | 151 | 158 | 164 | 171 | 177 | 184 | 190 | 197 | 203 | 210 | 216 | 223 | 230 | 236 | 243 | 249 | 256 |
| 69 | 128 | 135 | 142 | 149 | 155 | 162 | 169 | 176 | 182 | 189 | 196 | 203 | 209 | 216 | 223 | 230 | 236 | 243 | 250 | 257 | 263 |
| 70 | 132 | 139 | 146 | 153 | 160 | 167 | 174 | 181 | 188 | 195 | 202 | 209 | 216 | 222 | 229 | 236 | 243 | 250 | 257 | 264 | 271 |
| 71 | 136 | 143 | 150 | 157 | 165 | 172 | 179 | 186 | 193 | 200 | 208 | 215 | 222 | 229 | 236 | 243 | 250 | 257 | 265 | 272 | 279 |
| 72 | 140 | 147 | 154 | 162 | 169 | 177 | 184 | 191 | 199 | 206 | 213 | 221 | 228 | 235 | 242 | 250 | 258 | 265 | 272 | 279 | 287 |
| 73 | 144 | 151 | 159 | 166 | 174 | 182 | 189 | 197 | 204 | 212 | 219 | 227 | 235 | 242 | 250 | 257 | 265 | 272 | 280 | 288 | 295 |
| 74 | 148 | 155 | 163 | 171 | 179 | 186 | 194 | 202 | 210 | 218 | 225 | 233 | 241 | 249 | 256 | 264 | 272 | 280 | 287 | 295 | 303 |
| 75 | 152 | 160 | 168 | 176 | 184 | 192 | 200 | 208 | 216 | 224 | 232 | 240 | 248 | 256 | 264 | 272 | 279 | 287 | 295 | 303 | 311 |
| 76 | 156 | 164 | 172 | 180 | 189 | 197 | 205 | 213 | 221 | 230 | 238 | 246 | 254 | 263 | 271 | 279 | 287 | 295 | 304 | 312 | 320 |
| BMI | 19 | 20 | 21 | 22 | 23 | 24 | 25 | 26 | 27 | 28 | 29 | 30 | 31 | 32 | 33 | 34 | 35 | 36 | 37 | 38 | 39 |

# Preparation

## Your Target Weight Loss and Weight Loss Rate

The next step is to choose the rate at which you want to lose weight. You can choose a rate of half, one, two, or three pounds per week. Subtract you current weight from your target weigh. Then use the following table to help you identify how long it will take you to get to the target according to your chosen weekly weight loss rate.

| Pounds lost per week target | 0.5 | 1 | 2 | 3 |
|---|---|---|---|---|
| Calories lost per week target | 1750 | 3500 | 7000 | 10500 |
| Calories lost per day Target | 250 | 500 | 1000 | 1500 |
| Weigh loss target in pounds | Weeks to reach target | | | |
| 20 | 9 | 4 | 2 | 1 |
| 30 | 14 | 6 | 3 | 1 |
| 40 | 19 | 9 | 4 | 2 |
| 50 | 23 | 11 | 5 | 2 |
| 60 | 28 | 13 | 6 | 3 |
| 70 | 33 | 15 | 7 | 3 |
| 80 | 37 | 17 | 8 | 4 |
| 90 | 42 | 19 | 9 | 4 |
| 100 | 47 | 22 | 10 | 5 |
| 110 | 51 | 24 | 11 | 5 |
| 120 | 56 | 26 | 12 | 6 |
| 130 | 60 | 28 | 13 | 6 |
| 140 | 65 | 30 | 14 | 7 |
| 150 | 70 | 32 | 15 | 7 |

## Energy Balance Targets

The next step is to establish your Estimated Energy Requirement Target (EERT). Use the following table to choose it. Circle the EERT value that corresponds to your age range and you sex. For this purpose, we are assuming a value corresponding to a sedentary lifestyle. If that is not the case for you, use the value corresponding to your activity level (moderate or active) on the table.

| Female Estimated Energy Requirement Targets | | | |
|---|---|---|---|
| Age Range | Sedentary | Moderate | Active |
| 9-13 | 1600 | 1900 | 2200 |
| 14-18 | 1800 | 2100 | 2400 |
| 19-30 | 2000 | 2200 | 2400 |
| 31-50 | 1800 | 2000 | 2200 |
| 51+ | 1600 | 1900 | 2200 |
| Male Estimated Energy Requirement Targets | | | |
| Age Range | Sedentary | Moderate | Active |
| 9-13 | 1800 | 2200 | 2600 |
| 14-18 | 2200 | 2700 | 3200 |
| 19-30 | 2400 | 2700 | 3000 |
| 31-50 | 2200 | 2600 | 3000 |
| 51+ | 2000 | 2400 | 2800 |

Congratulations! Your key targets are now established. You know how much you should lose, how much you want to lose per week, and how low long it should take you to lose it. You will refer to this information later when you start to devise you daily food intake and physical activity plans.

You can now move on to the next section to start developing your strategy to help you accomplish the goal.

## Step 2 - Develop Your Strategy

This step will help you develop a strategy to accomplish your targets.

The Fitness Improvement Strategy Framework

Improving your fitness will require that you accomplish the following three things:

- Adjust and manage your lifestyle.
- Adjust and manage your nutrition.
- Adjust and manage your physical activity.

Let us explore some good reasons why these are so critical to your success and what the strategy should contain:

You should adjust and manage your lifestyle because the way you have been living has led to your current fitness condition. If you continue to do the same things, you will most likely continue to get the same results. Your strategy should include efforts to resolve the root cause(s) or top reason(s) why you have not been eating right, and have not been active enough. Moreover, this strategy should include efforts to help you adjust and manage conditions, situations, moods, and habits that affect your fitness.

You should adjust and manage your nutrition because the amount and type of food you eat affects calories and nutrients you ingest. As with your approach to life, if you carry on the same approach you will not make any progress in this critical aspect. Your strategy should include effort to improve the quality and nutritional balance of food you eat and reduce caloric intake, at least until you reach your target BMI. Once achieved, you should start to maintain energy balance to maintain your fitness level.

You should adjust and manage your physical activity because the amount and type of your daily physical activity affects how many calories you burn, your cardiovascular capacity, physical strength and flexibility, your agility, and so on. Continuing to stay at your current activity level will not lead to any progress. A sound fitness-improvement strategy requires both physical activity as well as nutritional adjustments. Your strategy should include efforts to improve cardiovascular capacity, strength, and flexibility.

The most effective fitness improvement strategy would be one developed in full alignment with the basic fitness principles and guidelines presented in prior sections. To help accomplish such alignment, we have developed a framework involving the following four action categories:

- Things you should eliminate, get rid of, throw away, stop doing, etc.
- Things you should add, obtain, buy, start doing, etc.
- Things you should increase, seek, accelerate, maximize, do more of, etc.
- Things you should reduce, avoid, do less of, etc.

Fitness Strategy Alignment

The figure on the next page shows the results of the alignment process. In it, you can easily see each of the key fitness principles and guidelines aligned to one of the four framework action categories and one of the three key strategy components. It provides a set of actions, which, if followed, should enable successful target achievement.

If you prefer a larger copy, you may download it from www.fitnessprotocols.com/book/forms.pdf.

# Fitness Improvement Strategy

| Action Categories | Lifestyle Adjustments | Nutrition Adjustments | Physical Activity Adjustments |
|---|---|---|---|
| **Eliminate, get rid of, throw away, stop doing, etc.** | Clean out bad foods from environments. | Eliminate junk food and high calorie drinks consumption. | |
| | Get rid of ALL clothing as soon as they become to large to wear. | | |
| | Start monitoring daily calories, weight, and activity. | Start eating on a consistent schedule. | Start completing 10000 steps a day. |
| **Add, get, buy, start doing, etc.** | Start following a fairly rigid weekly plan and schedule. | Start preparing food at home | Start building muscle mass. |
| | Display your commitment prominently were you can see it often. | Start bringing food with you when you leave the house | Start a balance activity program. |
| | | Start eating smaller more frequent well-balanced meals | Start stretching before physical activity. |
| | | Start reading food labels | Start learning and practicing basic Yoga moves. |
| | Avoid unsupportive environments. | Avoid mood altering drinks and food | Reduce time on non-active things. |
| **Reduce, minimize, avoid, do less, etc.** | Avoid unsupportive people. | Avoid becoming too hungry | |
| | Avoid mood altering conditions and situations. | Reduce mono unsaturated fat consumption | |
| | Avoid eating out. | Reduce simple carbohydrate consumption | |
| | | Reduce fatty-Protein consumption | |
| **Increase, accelerate, maximize, do more of, etc.** | | Increase water intake | Reduce injury risk by following a gradual physical activity plan. |
| | | Increase lean protein consumption | |
| | | Increase complex carbohydrates consumption. | |

The suggested strategy contains the broad set of guidelines you should adhere to in order to accomplish the targets you want to achieve.

In the next section, we will help you bring everything together into specific action plans and schedules. That will be the key to your success.

If you have done all the preparation work we have asked you to do, your plans will be comprehensive and will be highly useful to you as you delve into your new approach.

Now that you have targets and a broad strategy, you are ready to devise plans to help you accomplish the targets.

## Step 3 - Device Your Plans

This step will help you devise action plans to help you improve and maintain your fitness.

Devising Your Plans

This is the final and most critical step in the preparation protocol process as shown in the figure below.

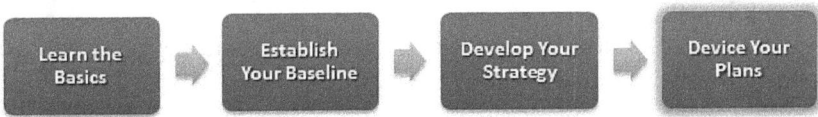

In this section, we will help you plan, organize, and set up your new approach to life, nutrition, and physical activity. As you saw in the strategy section, you need to do several things to enable your success. The focus is to help you actualize the actions necessary to reduce your weight by your chosen rate per week, and then help you keep it off once you successfully take it off. That is all this is! Here is where you will start taking advantage of the new knowledge you have acquired during the prior sections.

Four Key Plans

You need to devise four plans:

- Lifestyle Adjustment and Management Plan
- Nutrition Adjustment and Management Plan
- Physical Activity Adjustment and Management Plan
- The Set Up and Integration Plan

The Lifestyle Adjustment and Management Plan will help actualize your strategy for this aspect. It should include actions directed toward resolving the top reasons that led to your current condition, and actions to adjust and manage conditions, situations, moods, and habits that affect your fitness.

The Nutrition Adjustment and Management Plan will help you actualize your nutrition adjustment and management strategy. It should include action items that lead to improvement in the quality and nutritional balance of food you eat, and a reduction in caloric intake until you reach your target BMI.

The Physical Activity Adjustment and Management Plan will help you actualize your physical activity adjustment and management strategy. It should include action items that lead to improvement of your cardiovascular capacity, strength, and flexibility.

The Set Up and Integration Plan will help you get ready for success and prepare to integrate all these plans into your daily life.

**NOTE: This effort must become a top priority for a while. Nothing else should be more important! Otherwise, chances are your effort can fail-And you may end up being highly disappointed (perhaps again).**

## Plan 1 - Lifestyle Adjustment and Management Plan

This step will help you devise the plan to adjust and manage your lifestyle.

The Lifestyle Adjustment and Management Plan

This is a critical plan! The items included are critical to improving your fitness and remaining fit for life. Many get fit every year; however, few remain so for an extended period. Failing to make permanent adjustments to the way you live your life can be one of the main culprits. Especially early on, lifestyle adjustment and management are very important! That is why you need to spend time and effort to devise ways to accomplish the following:

- Staying away from mood-altering conditions, situations, food, and drinks.
- Staying away from high calorie food and drinks.
- Operating in controlled environments.
- Staying away from non-supportive people.
- Following strict eating and physical activity regimens and schedules consistently.
- Avoiding doing what you used to do that was not working.

Making these adjustments may seem hard at the beginning! Nevertheless, doing so is critical to your success. If you cannot overcome these challenges, you will find it hard to achieve sustainable fitness improvement. The good news, however, is that as time passes it should become much easier. If you are successful, you will not even notice, and sooner than you can imagine. As habits form, these adjustments will integrate into your lifestyle. You will not even remember what you previously used to do.

Moments of Choice

Every day we face the cycle shown by the figure on the following page multiple times. We have many options from which to choose regarding many aspects of life. You should keep in mind that the decisions we make have implications that go along with them-As often as possible, when confronted with a moment of choice, ask what happens if I do and what happens if I do not. Consider the implications of each choice you have. Use your imagination or memory. Remember what happened when you did something in the past and what the repercussions were.

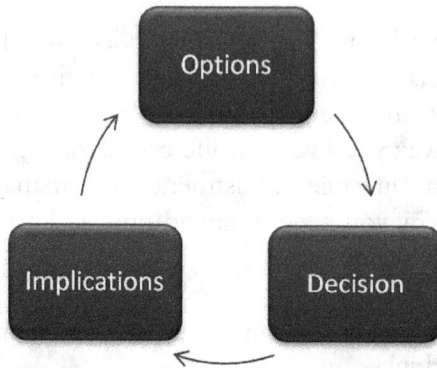

```
        ┌──────────┐
        │ Options  │
        └──────────┘
      ↗              ↘
┌──────────────┐   ┌──────────┐
│ Implications │   │ Decision │
└──────────────┘   └──────────┘
          ←
```

## The Biggest Challenges

The biggest challenges you will most likely face can manifest when you encounter conflicts between your goal and one of the following:

- Food you like to eat but is not good for you.
- People you like to be with but may not fully support your effort.
- Places you like to go to that offer poor choices.
- Situations you enjoy being in but can lead to making poor choices.
- Things you like to do that can distract you from being active.

Early on, avoidance may be the best strategy to follow for some of the above. Avoiding will be necessary only until your new habits form. Once that happens, your ability to manage these challenges will dramatically improve, lessening their emotional impact on you.

Preparation

Saying NO!

One of the key skills you need to develop is the ability of saying No! That means saying NO! to everything and everyone who does not support your effort. Here is where you need to use your commitment to help you muster high levels of courage and determination. A helpful technique you can use whenever you confront the need to say no is recalling the top reasons why you are doing this. If you want to aid your memory, refer the top list of the things you really do not want and the ones you want badly handy on pages 67 and 69. Those things led you down the path to improve your fitness so that you can live a better, more joyful life with those you care about most. In the end, they are what this is all for!

Giving in and Resilience

Realistically you will most likely give in to temptation here and there-It is human to do so. However, the world will not end because of it. If it happens, the most important thing to do is to bounce back. Do not allow a slip here or there to take you off track-off the main target-Try to be resilient. Therefore, if you fall off the horse, try getting back on it quickly and riding it again. You may find it useful to take a minute, after a mishap, to learn from the experience. Try to determine if there is any-thing you can do differently to avoid "falling off" next time.

Action Plan

We suggest you spend some time thinking about and choosing a few of the items you feel might be hardest for you to deal with from the following list:

- Staying away from mood-altering conditions, situations, food, and drinks.
- Staying away from high calorie food and drinks.
- Operating in controlled environments.
- Staying away from non-supportive people.
- Following strict eating and physical activity regimens and schedules consistently.
- Avoiding doing what you used to do that was not working.

If it comes up early on in the process, you should to come up with a quick action plan to deal with it. We have developed an easy form for you to use to document your plans if you wish to do so.

If you deem it necessary, use the form on the following page to develop a quick plan for any chosen item above. Make copies of the form before you start in case you need more than one.

If you prefer a larger copy, you may download it from www.fitnessprotocols.com/book/forms.pdf.

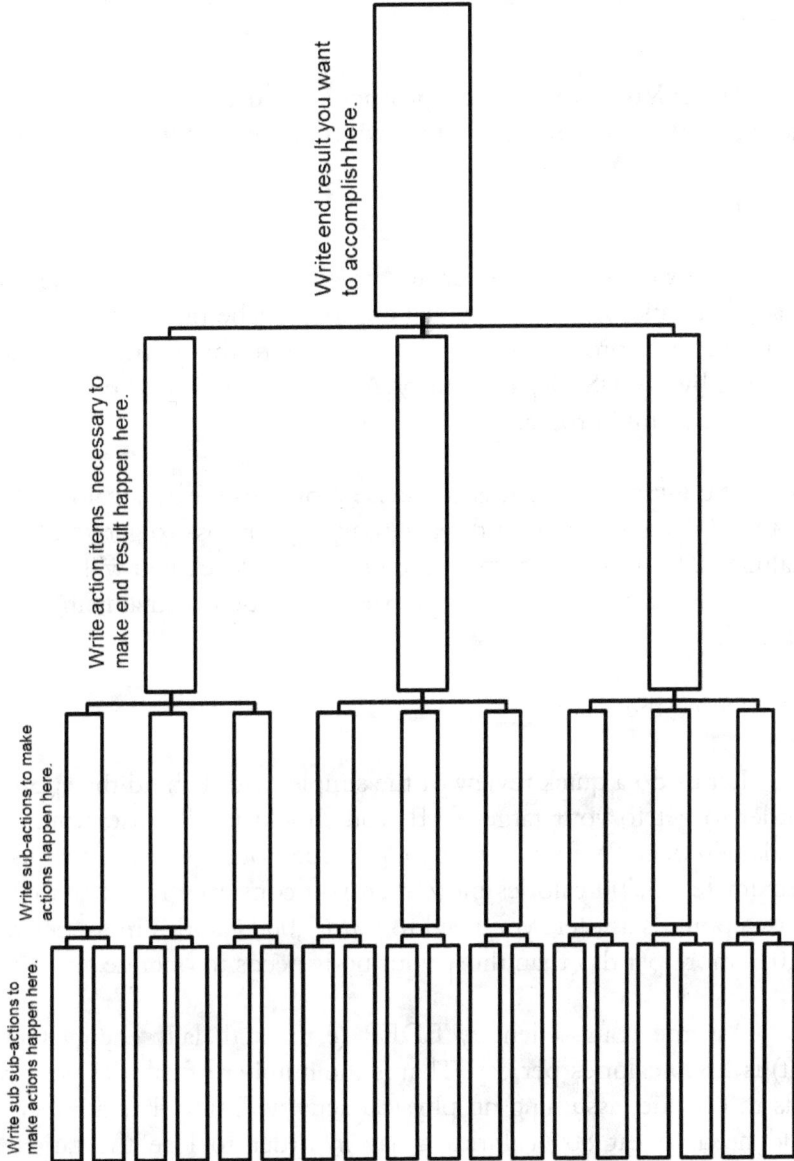

Write end result you want to accomplish here.

Write action items necessary to make end result happen here.

Write sub-actions to make actions happen here.

Write sub sub-actions to make actions happen here.

## Plan 2 - Nutritional Adjustment and Management Plan

This step will help you devise the plan to adjust and manage your nutrition.

**Note: Visit www.fitnessprotocols.com for information about tablet apps that can make the following section easier to manage.**

The Planning Approach

Here we will help you create a plan to help you make the necessary adjustments to your nutritional approach. The nutrition recommendations we will provide you are based upon the nutritional science developed by the US Department of Agriculture and used on their well-known MyPyramid program.

The initial approach is to devise a plan to create a caloric imbalance to help you accomplish the necessary weight loss to get you back to a healthier BMI level. Once you reach the target level, you will then need to adjust the plan to create energy balance needed to maintain an ideal BMI level.

Doing the Math

Let us do a quick review of the simple math behind the approach. In order to get to your target BMI, you should ideally lose around two pounds per week. We know that to lose one pound you need to use up approximately 3,500 calories more than you consume. In other word, to lose two pounds a week, you need to burn 7,000 calories more per week, or 1,000 more per day than those your body needs to operate.

Assume your sedentary EDER (estimated daily energy requirement) is 1,800 calories per day. That is the number of calories your body needs to operate, assuming no physical activity. Using that number, you would need to eat 800 calories a day in order to lose the target two pounds a week. However, that would be hard to do and not very healthy. You could not get enough nutrients from such a low number of calories. If you recall, the best approach to fitness improvement requires both physical activity and nutritional adjustment. If that is the case, you should add daily physical activity calories to your energy balance equation to use up between 500 to 1,000 calories. By adding physical activity, you can now eat more food in order to obtain a more balanced nutrient intake.

Let us assume you use/burn an additional 800 calories by adding physical activities to your day. Also, assume that half of them are burned by your typical daily activities during the day and the other half come from planned physical exercise. Now we have 800 plus 1,800 or 2,600 calories. When you subtract the 1,000-calorie deficit you need to get to your BMI target, you end up getting a much more reasonable 1,600-calorie nutritional plan to devise.

The Nutrition Plan

Let us now start devising your own plan. If you recall, the nutritional strategy we recommended earlier to help adjust and manage your nutrition suggested you do the following:

- Reduce monounsaturated fat consumption.
- Reduce simple carbohydrate consumption.
- Reduce fatty-protein consumption.
- Start eating smaller, more frequent well-balanced meals.
- Increase lean protein consumption.
- Increase complex carbohydrates consumption.
- Increase water intake.

The plan we will help you produce will meet the aforementioned suggestions. The initial food intake plan we recommend for you will be a starting point. To make it work best, you should to try it out for a couple of weeks. Once you do, you can tweak it as you go to make it fit you best.

Use the following form to help you estimate how many calories you need to get from your daily food intake.

| Calorie Level Estimator | Yours | Example |
|---|---|---|
| Estimated Daily Energy Requirement (from Page 169) | | 2200 |
| Minus the Daily Caloric Deficit Target (from Page 168) | | 1000 |
| Plus Activity Calories Use Target (Estimated) | | 400 |
| Daily Food Intake Calorie Level (TOTAL) | | 1600 |

Based on the Daily Food Intake Calorie (TOTAL) you estimated above, use the table on the following page to help you determine your daily food intake by food group.

Notice there are actually two tables in one: one for the major food groups and one (at the bottom) that breaks up the vegetables up by their groups. This provides you more specificity.

Please note that you also get a number of discretionary calories to play with every day.

If you prefer a larger copy, you may download it from www.fitnessprotocols.com/book/forms.pdf.

# Preparation

| Calorie Level | | Daily Amount of Food From Each Group | | | | | | | | | | |
|---|---|---|---|---|---|---|---|---|---|---|---|---|
| | 1,000 | 1,200 | 1,400 | 1,600 | 1,800 | 2,000 | 2,200 | 2,400 | 2,600 | 2,800 | 3,000 | 3,200 |
| Food Groups | | | | | | | | | | | | |
| Cups of Fruit | 1 | 1 | 1.5 | 1.5 | 1.5 | 2 | 2 | 2 | 2 | 2.5 | 2.5 | 2.5 |
| Cups of Vegetable | 1 | 1.5 | 1.5 | 2 | 2.5 | 2.5 | 3 | 3 | 3.5 | 3.5 | 4 | 4 |
| Eq Oz of Grain | 3 | 4 | 5 | 5 | 6 | 6 | 7 | 8 | 9 | 10 | 10 | 10 |
| Eq Oz of Meat and Beans | 2 | 3 | 4 | 5 | 5 | 5.5 | 6 | 6.5 | 6.5 | 7 | 7 | 7 |
| Cups of Milk | 2 | 2 | 2 | 3 | 3 | 3 | 3 | 3 | 3 | 3 | 3 | 3 |
| Tsp of Oils | 3 | 4 | 4 | 5 | 5 | 6 | 6 | 7 | 8 | 8 | 10 | 11 |
| Total Calories from servings | 835 | 1029 | 1229 | 1468 | 1605 | 1733 | 1910 | 2038 | 2190 | 2374 | 2488 | 2552 |
| Discretionary Calories | 165 | 171 | 171 | 132 | 195 | 267 | 290 | 362 | 410 | 426 | 512 | 648 |
| Weekly Veggie Distribution | | | | | | | | | | | | |
| Calorie Level | 1,000 | 1,200 | 1,400 | 1,600 | 1,800 | 2,000 | 2,200 | 2,400 | 2,600 | 2,800 | 3,000 | 3,200 |
| Veggie Groups | | | | | | | | | | | | |
| Cups of dark green veggies per week | 1 | 1.5 | 1.5 | 2 | 3 | 3 | 3 | 3 | 3 | 3 | 3 | 3 |
| Cups of orange veggies per week | 0.5 | 1 | 1 | 1.5 | 2 | 2 | 2 | 2 | 2.5 | 2.5 | 2.5 | 2.5 |
| Cups of legumes per week | 0.5 | 1 | 1 | 2.5 | 3 | 3 | 3 | 3 | 3.5 | 3.5 | 3.5 | 3.5 |
| Cups of starchy veggies per week | 1.5 | 2.5 | 2.5 | 2.5 | 3 | 3 | 6 | 6 | 7 | 7 | 9 | 9 |
| Cups of other veggies per week | 3.5 | 4.5 | 4.5 | 5.5 | 6.5 | 6.5 | 7 | 7 | 8.5 | 8.5 | 10 | 10 |

These food groups and amounts should provide not only the targeted daily calories, but also deliver recommended well-balanced daily amounts of vitamins and minerals. We are going to provide you a wide-open set of food choices for you to choose in each of the categories above. In the next step we will help you will translate the broad plan above into more specific food choices, including a weekly eating schedule.

**NOTE: It is extremely important that you do the best you can to ensure the food choices you make are as much as possible within your food taste zone. If you choose food that is way outside, it may be much harder to make eating it part of your normal life! This one of the typical reasons many diets out there fail to stick.**

Nonetheless, we hope you keep an open mind when making your food selections. You would be amazed how much food you think you do not like until you try it. On the other hand, if you are certain about your dislike of a particular food, there can be many ways to prepare it to make it look and taste much better.

Be aware that we do not provide any food preparation suggestions here. We will leave that up to you.

Daily Food Choices and Schedule

Use the form on the following page to devise your weekly food intake plan according to the recommended amounts in the table on page 185 and based on your calorie target. You may want to make several copies of the form before you start. Please note you need a form for every meal per tabs on top of the form.

If you prefer a larger copy, you may download it from www.fitnessprotocols.com/book/forms.pdf.

Do not forget to transfer your eating schedule onto your smartphone or other personal scheduling system you use.

## Weekly Meal Food Intake Planner

| Day of Week | Meal Time | Cups of Vegetable | | | | | Cups of Fruit | Cups of Grain | Eq. Oz. of Protein | Eq. Oz. of Dairy | Tbs. of Oil |
| | | Dark Green | Orange | Starchy | Legumes | Other | | | | | |
|---|---|---|---|---|---|---|---|---|---|---|---|
| Monday | | | | | | | | | | | |
| Tuesday | | | | | | | | | | | |
| Wednesday | | | | | | | | | | | |
| Thursday | | | | | | | | | | | |
| Friday | | | | | | | | | | | |
| Saturday | | | | | | | | | | | |
| Sunday | | | | | | | | | | | |
| Recommended Portions | | | | | | | | | | | |
| Planned Portions | | | | | | | | | | | |
| Unplanned Portions | | | | | | | | | | | |

Meal times: Breakfast | Morning Snack | Lunch | Afternoon Snack | Dinner | Evening Snack 1 | Evening Snack 2

## Plan 3 - Physical Activity Adjustment and Management Plan

This step will help you devise the plan to adjust and manage your physical activity.

The Planning Approach

We will help you create a plan to help you make the necessary adjustments to your physical activity approach. If you recall from the prior plan, the initial approach is to create an imbalance that will lead to the weight reduction necessary to get you to a much healthier BMI level. You will have many alternatives to burn calories through physical activities. A well-balanced approach should include cardio, strength building, and flexibility-enhancing activities.

The Physical Activity Plan

Let us now start devising your own plan. If you recall, the strategy we recommended earlier to help adjust and manage your physical activity suggested you do the following:

- Reduce injury risk by following a gradual physical activity plan.
- Start learning and practicing basic Yoga moves.
- Start completing ten thousand steps a day.
- Start a balanced activity program.
- Start building muscle mass.
- Start stretching before physical activity.

The plan we will help you produce will meet the aforementioned suggestions. As with the nutrition plan, the initial recommendations we make for you will be a starting point. To make the plan work best, you should to try it out for a couple of weeks. Once you do, you can tweak it as you go to make it fit you best.

As you choose activities to burn calories, do not forget that physical activities provide a number of benefits beyond simply burning calories.

If you recall from the introduction, depending on the type, frequency, and intensity, physical activity can enhance your immune system, reduce stress, and build muscle mass. A stronger immune system can help prevent illnesses, reduce their chance of occurrence or duration, and mitigate their impact. Reduced stress has many benefits including the reducing the urge to eat due to stress-induced anxiety. Building muscle mass should help speed up your metabolism over time. A faster metabolism should make you burn more calories while you are at rest. You will also find that, if you do enough activity, you may be able to sleep much better and longer as a result.

Moreover, do not forget the potential for many other benefits such as more strength, flexibility, endurance, etc. Keep in mind that health benefits of physical activity increase with increasing levels of activity and do not plateau until quite high levels. Physical activity will be well worth the time and effort you put into it! Finally, we want to emphasize that many of these benefits should manifest quickly after you get going!

Physical Activity Choices and Schedule

We have designed an easy way for you to devise your physical activity plan. Use the table on Appendix A to choose activities based on the approximate amount of calories you are supposed to burn. You should select at least one activity in each of the three activity categories: cardio, strength, and flexibility. The idea is to start easy, slow, and work your way up as you build your physical capability. Your body will tell you when you are ready. If you like to push and go for it, just make sure you are capable of doing the activity and fit enough to embark on it.

**NOTE: Always check with your doctor or other credible medical authority to ensure you can indeed do what you want to do.**
With patience, you will get there in less time you think if all works out the way it should.

Please make sure to create a schedule that is realistic so that you can follow it consistently. There is nothing wrong with splitting your activities during the day.

The key is doing it-Start moving and burning more calories and other amazing benefits the activities will provide you over time.

One more important aspect is to start slow and easy. It takes time to get the body adjusted to physical activities. Do not try running a marathon in the first thirty days. Do not try to lift three hundred pounds of weights. Easy does it. Your body will tell you when to crank it up. Moreover, by taking it easy, you will avoid unnecessary pain and possibly injuries that can delay your effort and create excuses you do not need to have early on.

Finally, as with the food you choose to eat, make sure your activity choices are congruent with things you enjoy doing. If possible, find one or more physical activity friends or partners to work out with you. If you can afford it, seek professional help from a fitness coach. A coach can be very helpful to get you started on the right foot (no pun intended) and tune your activities so you can maximize your time and effort. Most local gyms have certified folks that can provide this service. The Web offers lots of advice, but you need to make sure you chose a credible source!

Daily Physical Activity Choices and Schedule

Use the form on the following page to devise your plan. You may want to make multiple copies of the form before you start.

If you prefer a larger copy, you may download it from www.fitnessprotocols.com/book/forms.pdf.

Preparation

| Activity Category | Session Time & Choice | Monday | Tuesday | Wednesday | Thursday | Friday | Saturday | Sunday |
|---|---|---|---|---|---|---|---|---|
| Cardio | Time 1 | | | | | | | |
| | Choice 1 | | | | | | | |
| | Time 2 | | | | | | | |
| | Choice 2 | | | | | | | |
| Strength | Time 1 | | | | | | | |
| | Choice 1 | | | | | | | |
| | Time 2 | | | | | | | |
| | Choice 2 | | | | | | | |
| Flexibility | Time 1 | | | | | | | |
| | Choice 1 | | | | | | | |
| | Time 2 | | | | | | | |
| | Choice 2 | | | | | | | |
| Recommended Calories | | | | | | | | |
| Planned Calories | | | | | | | | |
| Unplanned Calories | | | | | | | | |
| Recommended Steps | | | | | | | | |
| Equivalent Planned Steps | | | | | | | | |
| Equivalent Unplanned Steps | | | | | | | | |

**Weekly Physical Activity Planner**

Now that you have your daily plan set, you can move to develop your set up and integration plan. Do not forget to transfer your activity schedule onto your smartphone or other personal scheduling system you use.

## Plan 4 - Setup and Integration Plan

This step will help you devise the plan to set up and integrate.

Why Set up and Integration are Critical

The key to any successful strategy is the set up and integration process! Whatever your chosen approach is you must integrate it into your life and make it an important and integral part. Therein lays the secret to success and one of the primary reasons why many may fail to accomplish this important feat.

It is very important you recognize that setting up and integration are very important. Make sure to focus your energy on the effort to ensure it happens first thing. These plans and schedules you came up with earlier in the process are the vehicles to help you accomplish day-to-day integration. Thus, you should follow them accordingly.

Early on, one of the biggest challenges you could face might be overcoming the force of "old" routines and habits. This may be the case until you form new ones. The older you are and the longer you have been out of shape, the more challenging this could be.

Here is where your strong commitment, supported by the new knowledge you have acquired, will play a key role in mitigating these forces. A good integration plan will help further solidify these forces.

Your Top Priority and Primary Focus

As we have mentioned several times before, there should not be any competition to this effort!-It must become your sole focus-It needs to be your top and most critical priority until you are done. The good news is that as time passes and you make progress, this will become easier to accomplish. Eventually, if all goes well, it will take on a life of its own and you will not even need to think too much about it. It will feel more effortless. Your decision-making will become attuned to your new life-style, and your nutritional and physical activity approach. You will love and crave the (new) better food and physical activity. You will not need to think about it-It will feel effortless-It will feel awesome! Moreover, you will start feeling awesome too!

### The Setup and Integration Plan Aspects

This is a plan of the things you should do to get ready to start a new life-style and approach to nutrition physical activity.

There are three key aspects to creating this plan:

- Create a strategy-supportive schedule
- Establish supportive environments
- Get the things you need to get started

Let us go over a brief description of each of them:

### Create a strategy-supportive schedule

You should create and follow a master schedule to help you actualize your strategies and plans. The schedule translates plans into action. Having and following a rigid schedule is very important early on in the process. A schedule can help create habits. The schedule you create and follow should include all aspects of your life. It should also be fully congruent with your normal life cycle. If set too far off from your natural cycles, it may not stick. You need to become as consistent as possible about following your schedule. The good news, for those less structured, is that as things become habitual you will have less of a need for so much formality. Nevertheless, early on, high structure is essential!

### Establish supportive environments

You should establish supportive environments before you start doing anything else. As we have mentioned before, the environment is very important! Supportive environments enable your effort. You need to eliminate or mitigate temptation by ridding your key environments of all the food and drinks that do not support your new approach. This may be more challenging if you share your environment with others who are not following your approach or do not support your effort. Even then, you need to find a way to organize things such that your food and drinks are available and those items that may be tempting to you in a weak moment are as much out of sight as possible. This can be critical early on!

Get the things you need to get started

You should identify and get ahold of all the things you need to get started. This includes any professional advice or support, memberships in clubs, clothing and fitness apparel, food, food preparation items, supplements, fitness equipment and gear, and any learning material and references. Everything should be in place if possible to start. There should be nothing missing-Not having some of these items may provide excuses for skipping or missing important action per your plans. Be ready-Try to have everything you need on day one!

## The Setup and Integration Plan

Create a strategy-supportive schedule

The good news is that you have completed most of the scheduling work already. All you need to do is to add a few more items that are important. The items you need to schedule are weekly time slots you should set aside to accomplish the following key weekly tasks:

- Maintain your environments.
- Plan and schedule the next week.
- Do food shopping.
- Prepare and precook food for next week.
- Review progress and make adjustments.

These will most likely end up as recurring tasks you will accomplish week after week at the same or similar time depending on your situation. Please take a minute to schedule these recurring items on you scheduling system.

Establish your supportive environments

In order to establish supportive environments, you need to accomplish the following tasks:

- Organize and clean your environments.
- Eliminate bad food and drinks from your environments.
- Display commitment certificate prominently.
- Verify you have enough food items available on your schedule.
- Verify you have all the necessary food preparation items available.

You should add these items to your schedule also. In addition, you should review them on a regular basis, especially if there are other people involved who affect your environments.

Environments include your home, work, and car. The place you live in is the primary environment of most concern. Inside the home, you need to focus on cleaning, organizing, and managing the pantry and other food storage cabinets, the refrigerator, and freezer. Moreover, you need to make sure food preparation items such as pots and pans, dishes, storage containers, etc. are available, clean, ready, and easy to access when needed. Nothing can be more detrimental to the plan than not finding something you need or having to fumble through a bunch of junk to find what you need. Your focus needs to be on making the plan happen as smoothly as possible. The more pain you introduce, the higher the chance of not following through. As we have said before, you do not need any excuses. There will be plenty of challenges; try not to introduce any more if you can help it.

We recommend you take the following "clean sheet" approach to establishing your environments:

1. Empty out everything.
2. Sort out food and drinks per the good/bad recommendations.
3. Throw or give away, or set aside the items that do not fit your plans.
4. Inventory all cooking accessories and equipment.
5. Clean up spaces (food storage, refrigerator, etc.).
6. Organize the items in some logical order back in the empty clean space.

This process requires courage and determination. You need to muster as much of these two as you can. A clean and well-organized environment will make a huge difference! It is well worth your effort! It should be the first thing you do! As we said earlier, it may be more challenging if there are others involved. You need to work it out with them. They need to understand how important this is for you. You need to reach some type of agreement with them to ensure full cooperation. This will be critical only in the first couple of months of your effort at the most. The environment, while always important, should not be as much of a challenge for you once your new habits take hold.

Get the things you need to get started

Finally, you need to have all the things you need available at the onset. Make a list of the items you need to get, and then schedule time to get them right away. We offer the following list as a guide of things you should consider:

- Professional advice or support
- Memberships to fitness clubs
- Clothing and fitness apparel
- Food and drinks
- Food preparation and storage items
- Fitness equipment and gear
- Learning material and references

Congratulations! You should now be ready to move forward-ready to start your journey to much better fitness and health.

# Change

This protocol will help you improve your fitness and lay the foundation for maintaining it afterward.

About the Change Stage

Change is the third stage in the Fitness Protocol process as shown in the figure below.

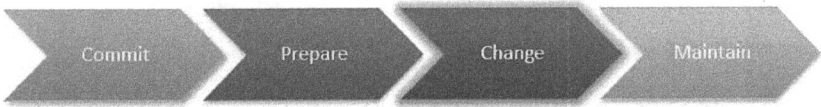

This is the stage where everything comes together to help you make fitness improvement a reality. Let us review what you have accomplished thus far:

- You made the decision to improve your fitness and developed a strong sense of commitment to do so.
- You learned everything you should know to support your effort.
- You established your fitness baselines and you set targets and devised plans to help you achieve them.

Accordingly, you should now be well prepared to make fitness improvement a reality! What remains is to follow through.

The Follow-Through Process

To help you follow through, we have devised the following five-step process illustrated by the figure below.

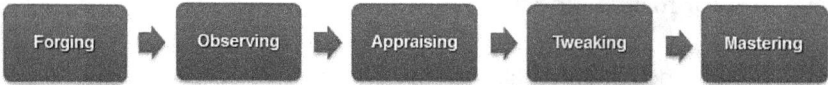

Forging → Observing → Appraising → Tweaking → Mastering

Each step in this process represents an activity you should complete in the sequence presented and on a routine basis until you reach your set fitness targets. Let us now review what each of these activities is:

Forging

Blacksmiths use heat and force to forge pieces of raw metal into more useful and better-looking objects. To accomplish their craft, they typically utilize a furnace to heat the metal, a heavy hammer, and an anvil to shape the metal. Moreover, they usually use a sketch or blueprint to guide them in their work.

This is a perfect metaphor for what you are about to do. In this case, you will become your own blacksmith and you are about to start the work to forge a better you. You will be using the commitment you have developed and knowledge you have acquired as your source of energy (heat and power) to accomplish the forging. Moreover, the targets you have set and the plans and schedule you have devised will serve as your blueprint.

Forging will most likely take a bit of time and effort to accomplish. There is significant work ahead of you. As with metal forging, forging the new and better you will require lots of energy, strength, and perseverance.

The forging activity simply involves following the plans and resulting schedule. Here you execute the tasks that will get you to eat better and become more physically active. As you follow these plans consistently, day in and day out, you will be forging habits that should make the initial effort much less so.

The Forging Process

The forging process is a critical one. Here is where your intentions meet your action. The following graphic shows the layers of accomplishments that have led you to this point.

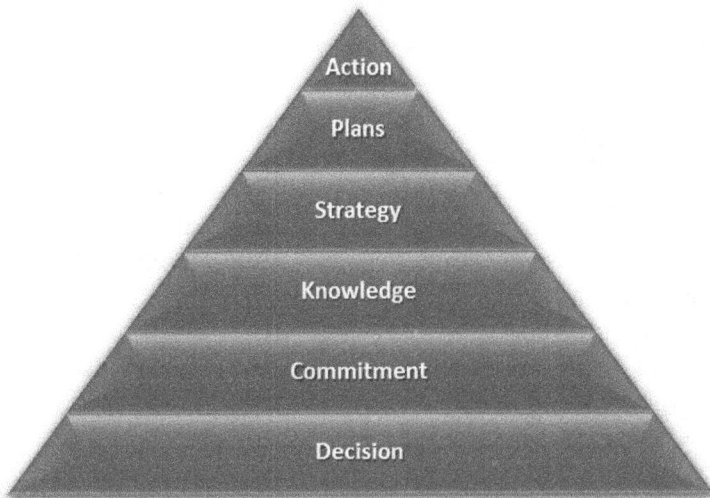

You started, at the bottom layer, by making the initial decision to improve your fitness. Then, you purchased this guide to help you with the process. We helped you build your commitment. We provided new knowledge. We helped you develop a strategy and devise the plans to make it happen. Now you are ready to take action.

Action is what the forging activity is about-It is all about doing it-It is about following the plans and schedules you devised to help accomplish what you set out to do. Forging is the first of five activities we suggest can help you follow through with your fitness improvement plans.

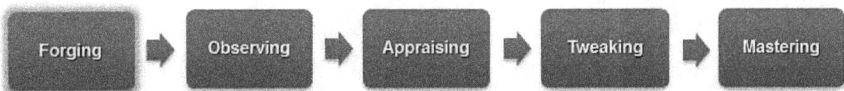

A successful forging process will require completed adjustment and management plans for your life-style, nutrition, physical activities, plus a set up and integration one. Also highly critical to this process will be creating, maintaining, and following a weekly master schedule that includes times and dates for nutrition, physical activity, and all other related tasks.

The forging process is about integrating you commitment, knowledge, and plans into your daily life.

**NOTE: The secret to successful integration is diligently setting, and consistently maintaining and following a master schedule. This effort needs to be a high priority. All activities aimed at improving your fitness MUST become your most important endeavor for a while. You need to be consistent about it. No deviations-No exceptions-It is critical!**

Forging Challenges

As we discussed in earlier sections, a number of things will most likely push you back during your effort to improve your fitness. These pushbacks, illustrated by the diagram bellow, run against the motivational force that the combination of your commitment and knowledge produces.

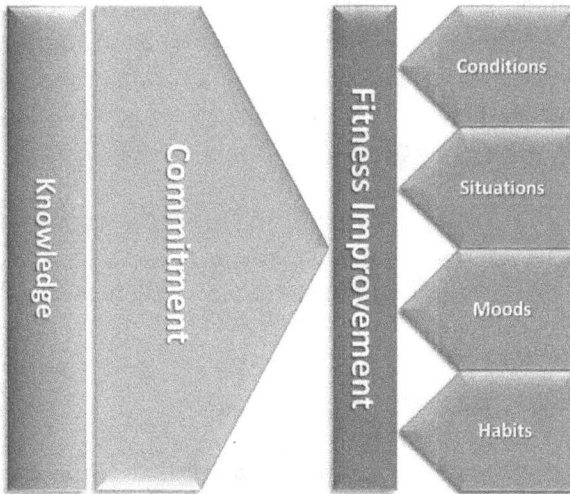

Moreover, as you start to form new habits, those new habits will transfer energy over to the left side and contribute additional energy to combat the others forces. Additionally, as you make progress and begin to see and feel the benefits of your effort, additional force will transfer over to the left side, further enhancing your motivational forces. Nonetheless, the initial force produced by some of the pushbacks will require a lot out of you.

The stronger your commitment and knowledge, the easier it will be for you to counter the forces of the pushbacks. However, we do not want you to take any chances at this critical juncture. Therefore, we want to provide you with additional knowledge and skills to further ensure you are as ready as you can be to deal with some of the biggest challenges you may face.

**NOTE: We ask you to please pay extremely close attention to the information we are about to share with you. Doing so can have a significant impact on your ability to get through the forging process with a lot less effort and pain.**

Of all the pushback forces, none will prove to be more challenging than the force of your current habits. Habits are repeating patterns that over time are "automated" by the brain. The brain does that in order to free up valuable capacity for other seemingly important things. We wake up in the morning and go through our day thinking and behaving in very similar predictable ways. We do so day in and day out. Habits can be organized into multiple categories. In the following section, we will cover two of the most important types.

The first of the types we want to go over are what we call the enabling habits. These types of habit are important because they affect other very important things we do as humans. There is a particular set of enabling habits we call cognitive capacities.

Cognitive Capacities

The executive system of the brain, located in the frontal lobes, is responsible for a number of important cognitive capacities. We have chosen it because it is highly relevant to your ability to forge most effectively. Following is a list and brief description for the most relevant ones:

- Response Inhibition - The capacity to think before we act.
- Emotional Control - The capacity to keep emotions in check.
- Task Initiation - The capacity to take timely action on tasks we need or want to do.
- Planning & Prioritization - The capacity to plan and prioritize action in pursuit of a goal.
- Organization is the capacity to organize according to a system.
- Time Management - The capacity to comply with scheduled tasks, events, commitments, etc.
- Goal-Directed Persistence - The capacity to persist and overcome challenges and obstacles to achieve a goal.
- Flexibility - The capacity to modify plans as conditions and circumstances change.
- Metacognition - The ability to recognize and reflect upon one's own approach, behavior, performance, etc.

- Stress Tolerance - The ability to handle stressful situations and conditions without performance degradation.

According to research conducted by Chuck Martin, Richard Guare, PhD, and Peg Dawson, EdD, and published in their book SMARTS, most of us have three or four strong capacities or skills, as they call them, and three or four weak ones. In the book, they pose that once past a certain age just after our brains reach maturity; these capacities become set and are more difficult, if not impossible to change. Moreover, they suggest that because they are so hard to change, we should focus our attention on using our strongest capacities and devising ways to make up for our weakest ones.

As you can see, these capacities are important to your effort because the weak ones can present challenges beyond habit forging. For example if you were to have a weak capacity to plan and prioritize, you may have a hard time with a critical aspect of our proposed strategy of weekly planning and prioritizing. If you have a weak capacity to recognize your own behavior, you may not be able to evaluate your performance to plan on a weekly basis as we recommend. If you have a weak capacity for goal-directed persistence, you may end up giving up at the first few signs of inevitable challenges.

Given the potential impact these weak capacities can have, we highly recommend you spend time to identify your weakest ones. Doing so can help you to mitigate any effect they may have on your forging process. To help you do that, we have developed a simple self-evaluation form you can use to get a quick idea. However, if you wish to be more thorough about it, you can buy the book and get access to a more complete assessment. Regardless, we highly recommend that you identify them, one way, or the other.

**NOTE: Keep in mind that we all have strong and weak points. The key is to know and accept what they are, and to take full advantage of our strongest capacities and manage around our weaker ones. The ones in between the strong and weak ones do not seem to matter as much, according to the experts.**

Use the form on the following page to get a quick sense of your strongest and weakest capacities. Rate each capacity using a "1-10" scale. A "10" stands for your strongest and a "1" for the weakest ones.

If you prefer a larger copy, you may download it from www.fitnessprotocols.com/book/forms.pdf.

| Executive System Capacities | Level |
|---|---|
| Emotional Control: The capacity to keep your emotions in check | |
| Task Initiation: The capacity to take timely action on tasks you need or want to do | |
| Planning/Prioritization: The capacity to plan and prioritize action in pursuit of your goals | |
| Organization: The capacity to organize according to a system | |
| Time Management: The capacity to comply with scheduled tasks, events, commitments, etc. | |
| Goal-Directed Persistence: The capacity to persist and overcome challenges and obstacles to achieve a goal | |
| Flexibility: The capacity to modify plans as conditions and circumstances change | |
| Metacognition: The capacity to recognize and reflect upon your approach, behavior, performance etc. | |
| Stress Tolerance: The capacity to handle stressful situations and conditions without performance degradation | |

## Working Around Your Weakest Capacities

Now that you have identified your potentially weakest capacities, take some time to assess how each of them may affect your effort to improve your fitness. Once you have that, you can then devise ways to mitigate or eliminate their effect. Following are a few general suggestions for approaches you could employ if some of these capabilities are a weakness of yours.

- Emotional control: Avoid situations that can trigger strong emotions. Start by keeping track of words, situations, and people who tend to trigger these types of emotions and devise ways to avoid them, at least for a while. If you wish to get deeper into it, you can explore the meaning you are assigning what you see or hear to determine if it really is worth it.

- Task Initiation: Get help from technology or people. Set up reminders, alarms, etc. on your phone, computer, PDA, etc. On the other hand, have family or friends e-mail, text, call, tweet you, etc. to remind you of an action you need to take. If you can, delegate some of the tasks to others.

- Planning/Prioritization: Also, get help from technology or people. We have provided quite a planning capability in this app. However, you need to use it. Sitting down with others who may be better at this task is also a good strategy.

- Organization: Get help from others. Get help from the most organized person you know to get your environment ready. Bring the person back occasionally to help you ensure you do not lose organization. You can also hire a professional organizer to help you create and then follow a system. You can readily find these types of folks on the Web.

- Time Management: Here is another area where you can get help from technology or people. Set up reminders, alarms, etc. on your phone, computer, PDA, etc. On the other hand, have family or friends e-mail, text, call, tweet you, etc. to remind you of tasks you need to complete.

- Goal-Directed Persistence: Here you need to rely on the commitment you made. You need to keep it in front of you and refresh yourself on the commitment process you followed at the beginning. Continue to remember the reasons why you want to improve your fitness. The things you want to get away from and the things you wish to obtain from being more fit. That is the best source of energy you can find to get you back in the game. We all have moments of doubt. We all have bad days. The key to keep us persevering is the reason why we started this in the first place.

- Flexibility: The reality is that the plans you devised will most likely change along the way. That is why we have included a tweaking step as part of the process. Eventually, and sooner than you may think, things will become stable and your need to be flexible will be less. When you find yourself struggling with change, consider exploring the underlying reason why it is so hard. Ask yourself what can happen if you do and what can happen if you do not. That may help you flex a little.

- Metacognition: If you determine you have a hard time discerning how you are doing, consider getting feedback from others with whom you have developed a strong rapport and trust. Ask them to keep an eye on you and to point out specific behaviors that may be detrimental to your effort. This action may require courage to listen and act on the feedback. However, it may be necessary.

- Stress Tolerance: Avoid conditions and situations that can trigger stress. Keep track of things causing you the most stress and do all you can to avoid them. If you wish to get deeper into it, categorize things to determine those under your control and those outside of it. Once you have time separated, you should consider not allowing things outside your control to bother you as much. Consider and reframe what they mean to you. For the ones that you control, develop a way to address them to reduce their potential effect on you.

We hope these brief workaround ideas can at least help you start dealing with some of your weaker capabilities so that they are not as much of an impediment to your progress as they may otherwise be.

Let us now move on to review the information about the next type of habit.

Well-Formed Habits

The second of the habit types we want to go over are what we call well-formed habits. These habits are the type that formed well and thus operate well outside our conscious awareness. These habits are persistent and much harder to change. These types of habits are more of the behavioral kind as opposed to the enabling ones we covered earlier.

Let us start with some of the theory behind habit formation and change. We will examine the most recent available theory about how long it takes to form habits and what it takes to do so. The idea is to give you a sense of the extent of time and the effort required to change and form new habits. To help you had better understand how habits work, we will start by going over some of the most recent theories behind habit formation and change. First, let us look at how long it may take.

Well-Formed Habits Take Much Longer to Form and Change

Automaticity is a measure of our ability to perform a task without requiring deliberate attention or mental effort.

210

Change

For years, the theory of habit change claimed that it took twenty-one days of consistent repetition to form a habit. However, recent research shows habit formation time could vary dramatically, taking an average of sixty-six days. It took participants in this particular study anywhere between eighteen to two hundred fifty-four days to reach a steady level of automaticity, mainly depending on task difficulty. Phillippa Lally, Cornelia H. M. van Jaarsveld, Henry W. W. Potts, and Jane Wardle conducted the research in England and published the results in the July 2009 edition of the European Journal of Social Psychology.

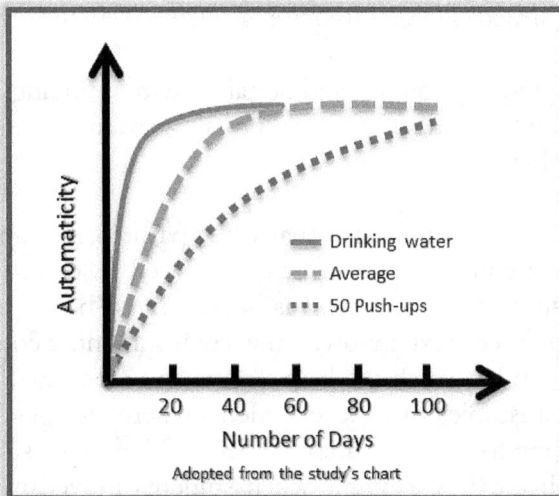

Adopted from the study's chart

The chart above shows that tasks that require less effort, such as drinking water on a daily basis, habituate more quickly. On the other hand, it shows that tasks requiring a lot more effort, such as doing fifty sit-ups a day, took much longer to habituate. One of the interesting and unexpected outcomes of this work points to the possibility that some of us may be more change-averse than others are. In this study, the more consistent the participants were at repeating the new behavior early on, the faster the behavior became automatic.

Following are the most relevant takeaways from this research concerning how long it takes to change or form habits:

1. It can take an average of two months, or so, to form a new habit.
2. Some habits can take longer to change than others.
3. Consistent repetition can help accelerate habit formation.

Now that you have a better sense of how long it can take, and of some possible ways to accelerate formation, we will look at what it takes to do so.

Well-Formed Habits Require a Diligent Effort to Form and Change

Before moving on to additional research findings from other sources, we want to share two additional relevant findings from the aforementioned study.

First, the results indicated that when participants repeated behaviors in consistent contexts, automaticity increased following a predictable pattern. This suggests that context is important to habit formation and change. A habit's context involves the environment, people, situation, and conditions under which the habit forms and reoccurs. Similar results were obtained in studies of college students where changes in conditions caused by moving to a new location helped or hindered a student's ability to maintain a habit. For example when students moved to a new place where they did not have easy access to exercise equipment, they stopped doing exercise.

Second, the results indicated, "missing one opportunity to perform the behavior did not materially affect the habit formation."

Now we will move on to additional research led by Professor Wendy Wood, currently working at the University of Southern California. This research is the most extensive and relevant research on habit change and formation we have uncovered. According to published records, Professor Wood and a number of her colleagues have been conducting habit research since 1998.

The most recent work on the subject available from Wood and colleagues Quinn, Pascoe, and Neal, sheds light on what it really takes to change well-formed or stubborn habits. Let us start by first reviewing their key findings:

*Participants in our studies were reasonably successful at exerting control over unwanted responses when they used self-control strategies that are tailored to the specific cuing mechanisms that produced the response (i.e., temptations vs. habits). Thus, as suggested in earlier research on delay of gratification, having sufficient control strength is not a guarantee of successful control. The participants in our diary and laboratory studies were most successful when they exerted control in ways best suited to inhibiting the habit mechanism that activated the unwanted response.*

*Motivation of course plays an important role in self-control. People change responses when they intend to do so and when they believe they have the efficacy to perform an alternative response. However, simply being motivated does not ensure that people will overcome effectively the conflicting automatic triggers in performance environments. Such exertion of self-control requires control over the automatic, undesired response to the cue.*

*We were able to show that, although vigilant monitoring of behavior is not useful for temptations, it is an especially effective form of self-control for habits. Because habit responses are activated in memory upon perception of associated context cues, the challenge for habit control is to inhibit tendencies to perform that activated response (Neal et al., 2009). Careful monitoring for unwanted responses provided this control over habits. Distraction proved somewhat counterproductive, which is understandable given that unwanted habits are especially likely to be cued by triggering stimuli when people's attention is otherwise engaged (Reason, 1992).*

*We speculate that effortful inhibition contributes most productively to behavior change when the suppression of undesired responses is paired with learning and performing a new, desired response. That is, inhibition might be effective as a short-term strategy to suppress an unwanted habit so as to enable a new, more desired pattern of responding to be established. If the new response is repeated in contiguity with context cues, then new good habits might be formed. For example, a dieter's effortful inhibition of unhealthful eating habits may promote long-term behavior change only insofar as it creates a temporary window of opportunity in which to establish healthful eating patterns. In this view, the inhibition of cued responding is a short-term means of control that, although perhaps inherently unsustainable in itself, enables the development of new, more desired patterns of response consistent with goals. One limit to this process is that, when newly learned associations override older ones (e.g., extinction), the new learning is inherently unstable such that the original learning may readily recur under a variety of circumstances (Bouton, 2000). This spontaneous recurrence is one feature of habits that makes them difficult to change. Nonetheless, the monitoring strategy that we identified in the present investigation provides an initial handle on the challenge of altering unwanted habits.*

Following are the most relevant takeaways from both research studies concerning what it takes to form and/or change habits:

1. Repeating habits under consistent conditions can accelerate habit formation.
2. Skipping practice occasionally may not impede ultimate habit formation.
3. Vigilant monitoring of your behavior can be an effective method of self-control for habits.
4. Paying close attention to what triggers a habit can be an effective approach.
5. Suppressing unwanted habits can work as long as it is done in conjunction with forming a new habit.
6. Motivation alone does not ensure you can overcome the automatic mechanisms behind some of your habits.

As you may be able to conclude from the preceding information, habits can be a force to be reckoned with. Changing some of your older well-formed habits and forming new ones may not be easy. It will require high levels of commitment and motivation and careful attention to what triggers them. Moreover, it will also require a good dose of both patience and perseverance to see you through the number of months of effort that they may take to change or form.

The strategies and tools that we provide to you here are designed with the challenge in mind. We strongly recommend you adhere to our suggestions to help you manage one of the most significant challenges you can face in the process of improving your fitness.

The Enabling Routines

There are number of activities that can make a big difference. These are what we consider to be high-leverage activities because they enable other activities downstream. When you complete them, they set up your ability to get something else done. We call these activities enabling routines.

The following list shows the five key enabling routines we highly recommend you consistently complete once a week at a minimum:

- Maintain your environments.
- Plan and schedule the following week.
- Do food shopping.
- Prepare and precook food for next week.
- Review progress and make adjustments.

Completing these routines will enable you to adhere to the critical daily activities that will ultimately lead to improved fitness. Therefore, you need to work as hard as possible to ensure these weekly routines happen. They really are the key to your success!

That means time for these routines needs to be a high priority on your weekly schedule. Week in and week out, you must ensure the following:

- That you take time to ensure your key environments support your effort.
- That you take time to plan and schedule the upcoming week.
- That you take time shopping, preparing, and precooking food per your plan.
- That you have the right food available at the right time.
- That you take time to observe, assess progress, and tweak your plans if necessary.

Excuses Galore

Here is a list of some classic excuses we all use to justify not completing some of our fitness-related activities:

- I did not have (enough) time
- I ran out of...
- I forgot...
- I did not have...
- I was in a bad mood
- I was not in the mood
- I was stressed out
- I was hungry
- I could not say NO!
- I did not feel like it
- I did not have another/better option
- I had something come up

Sometimes these will be legitimate reasons for a mishap here and there. However, most of the time the reasons we come up with are just excuses. The real problem can be that when using excuses perpetuates ending up derailing your fitness improvement effort. Attention to this matter becomes especially important if you recognize and acknowledge you are becoming a habitual excuse-maker. Regardless of whether you are becoming one or not, the best strategy for debunking excuses is focusing your attention and effort on the completion of the enabling routines covered earlier. Doing so will make things seem a lot easier to do, without the need to resort to excuse making.

Building Momentum

It may take a little bit of time to find your stride. However, in order to find it you need to get started first. One of the basic laws of physics tells us "objects at rest tend to remain at rest and objects in motion tend to remain in motion."

Once you start moving, you can build momentum. As momentum builds, your efforts will require a lot less emotional energy to keep you moving. Motion will lead to progress and as you make more progress, it will reinforce you and keep your momentum going. Your weight will start to come off. The inches will start shedding. Your energy will start to rise. You will start feeling stronger. Moreover, you will start to look and feel better-Momentum builds even more.

Unless something major gets in the way, you will never stop. Your new habits will become unconscious to you. Your daily and weekly routines will seem second nature. You will actually miss them if you skip them for some reason. Getting back on the horse will be a lot easier if you were to fall off. It will be awesome!

Now that you have a better sense of the forging process, let us go over the observing process.

Observing

Observing is an important activity because you will be doing many new things. By paying close attention to them, you will make sure they are working well for you. Observing involves daily tracking of nutrient and caloric intake, body weight, physical activity, and a few other parameters. The information you gather will provide important and useful information you will in turn use to appraise your progress and tweak your effort if necessary.

The Observing Process

Significant evidence shows that regular observation is an essential element of successful fitness improvement strategies. Observing is the second activity we recommend to help you integrate the new approach into your life.

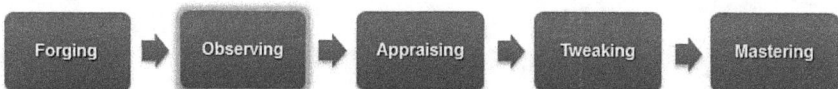

Forging ➡ Observing ➡ Appraising ➡ Tweaking ➡ Mastering

Make and log observations to help heighten awareness of the things that are working and of those that are not. These days observing has become a lot easier thanks to technology advances. We have provided a set of forms to help you keep track of progress within this guide. However, alternative tools for this purpose abound. Following we provide a description of some of what is available for your consideration.

Tools for Observing

One of the unique and best fitness monitoring and tracking tools we are aware of is the BODYMEDIA Fit System. The system consists of an armband monitor and an optional Web-based software service. The system monitors and keeps track of a number of fitness-related metrics including calories you burn, sleeping patterns, steps, and nutritional intake. Also available is a free iPhone app that allows you to see your data once you downloaded from the armband onto the Web site.

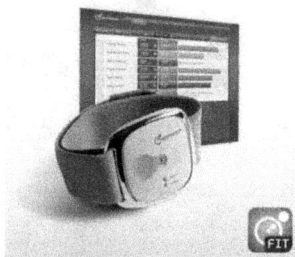

The system is highly accurate, easy to use, and is seamless to wear. It takes quite a bit of the work involved in observing and tracking off your hands. It is the ideal tool if you can afford it. Otherwise, there are many other tools and apps available out there, that cost less and can provide you with useful information. For example, pedometers can be a very useful tool to keep track of your daily steps. You can buy one for very little money or you can download an iPhone application such as "Pedometer" that enables the iPhone to act as one.

In case you wish to consider other alternatives, following are some iPhone apps that help track walking and running outdoors. The list ranks the apps as essential or notable, according to the AppGuides iPhone app as of the book writing:

Essential Apps:

- Nike+ GPS
- MotionX GPS
- Runmeter GPS Running

Notable Apps:

- AllSport GPS
- GPS Kit
- RunnKeeper
- Trailhead
- NB TotalFit

Following are some iPad apps for tracking food intake ranked the same way, according to the AppGuides iPhone app:

Essential Apps:

- MyNetDiary
- Calorie Counter

Notable Apps:

- Food Scanner
- GoMealsHD
- Diet and Fitness Tracker

Regardless of the way you choose to do it, we highly recommend you are as observant as possible early on in this process, ideally, until you reach your target. We strongly recommend that you closely track and observe your nutrient and caloric intake, your weight, your physical activity, and, if possible, your state of mind or mood.

The information you gather during your observation effort will provide important and useful feedback for you.

Now that you have a better sense of the observing process, let us go over the appraising process.

Appraising

The initial plans you devised are just a guide to get you started with your new approach. Therefore, they will most likely require some adjustment or tweaking. During the weekly appraisal process, you will review and analyze the information collected during the observation step. In this step, you will evaluate the effectiveness of your approach and if necessary make adjustments accordingly.

The Appraising Process

We recommend you analyze the information gathered during your observations on a regular basis. This appraisal should yield valuable intelligence you can use to make adjustments as you go. Remember that the plans you devised are just a guide. It is highly likely you will have to tweak them and do so often until you find your best approach. Appraising is the third activity we recommend to help you integrate the new approach into your life.

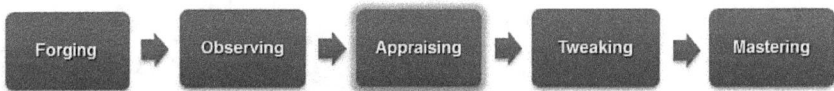

Forging ➡ Observing ➡ Appraising ➡ Tweaking ➡ Mastering

We recommend you complete a quick appraisal on a daily basis, and a more comprehensive one every week.

During daily appraisal, you should take a few minutes to appraise your day. You can do this right after you complete logging your observations for the day. The daily appraisal consists of answering a set of simple questions about follow-through, pushbacks, and the results you are getting from your effort. This effort can be highly valuable because it enables you to identify necessary adjustments earlier.

Change

During weekly appraisal, you should take the time necessary to appraise the aspects of your strategy, plans, and schedules that are working and those that are not. Your daily nutritional and physical activity efforts should produce sustainable weight loss and habit change. That means that if things are working as they should you should be losing weight at or near your weekly target rate. Moreover, you should also start feeling less and less tension between your old and new habits as time passes. Successful habit change and formation are critical because it is what will ultimately enable you to remain fit after you reach your target. That is the main reason for paying close attention to weekly weight loss and habit change and formation.

Be aware that is usual to run into weeks when your weight may not change, when it may increase a little, or when you may drop a "bunch" more than planned. Weight loss does not necessarily follow a perfect straight-line path. Nevertheless, if your weight is not coming down at all, is not coming down enough, or it is actually increasing, during a period longer than two weeks, you need to do something to effect change.

Following are some of the questions you should to seek answer when that happens:

- Are there things I should eliminate, get rid of, throw away, stop doing, etc.?
- Are there things I should add, obtain, buy, start doing, etc.?
- Are there things I should increase, seek, accelerate, maximize, do more of, etc.?
- Are there things I should reduce, avoid, do less of, etc.?

Now that you have a better sense of the appraising process, let us go over the tweaking process.

Tweaking

In this step, you will take what you learned from appraising the observed information and use it to adjust your plans as necessary. Tweaking will likely be an ongoing process. You learn as you go and you adjust as necessary.

The Tweaking Process

Tweaking is the fourth activity of the follow-through process we recommended for you.

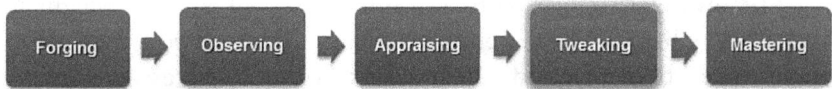

Forging ➡ Observing ➡ Appraising ➡ Tweaking ➡ Mastering

Here is when you will use the knowledge you gained after appraising the observations made while forging the plans you devised. As we have mentioned a number of times, the original plans were meant to get you started. Once you do, you will most likely need to adjust or tweak your plans based on emerging conditions and circumstances. This is the case with almost any plans devised for any purpose. As someone once said, "things never go according to plan." Tweaking should be an ongoing process. There will most likely be something to adjust all the time. As with appraising, you will most likely need to do some tweaking on a daily and weekly basis.

Now that you have a better sense of the forging tweaking, let us go over the mastering process.

Mastering

Mastering is the fifth and final activity of the follow-through process we recommended for you.

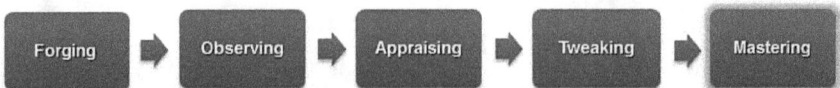

Forging ➡ Observing ➡ Appraising ➡ Tweaking ➡ Mastering

Mastery results from practice. Practice is all about repetition. Practice is a process that involves trial and error. Trial and error are essential aspects for mastery. Anyone who is achieving mastery of his or her craft practices a lot. Moreover, the person makes a lot of mistakes and corrections in the process. He or she is constantly forging, observing, appraising, and tweaking.

However, our aim is not to turn you into a "fitness master" per se. Our intention is to help you master yourself and your ability to create a fitness approach that yields sustainable fitness improvement. That is what you really need to master.

You will know when you have accomplished mastery when the following occurs:

- When conditions do not affect your fitness as much, or at all.
- When you do not have to avoid situations affecting your fitness anymore.
- When your mood does not get in the way of your fitness-related actions.
- When the tension you feel between old and new habits subsides.

The old pushbacks will be no more and you will feel in control of yourself and of your fitness. You will need to spend a lot less emotional energy to keep up the progress made. It will be a lot easier to bounce back from moods, conditions, or situations that get you off track. The tension you will feel will be more from the fitness activities you feel you "must" do. You will feel compelled to do physical activity and eating on schedule and eating right. That is what mastery should feel like.

We are aware that it may be hard for you to comprehend at this point, but soon, if you stick with it and follow the program, you will be able to feel it. You will be amazed!

Furthermore, empowered by the way you will look and feel when it happens, you will be much better able to master the rest of your life! The things you did not want in your life should be gone by then and those you wanted badly should be starting to appear if not there already.

## The Mastering Process

The mastering process is about mastering the process. "The process" is what should lead you to mastery. Following each of the steps in the process shown in the figure below should enable mastery.

The diagram on the following page shows a summary of the steps, activities, and their frequency. It shows a high-level view of what needs to be completed and how often at each stage.

If you prefer a larger copy, you may download it from www.fitnessprotocols.com/book/forms.pdf.

# Follow-Through Steps, Activities, and Frequencies

| Process Steps | Forge | Observe | Appraise | | Tweak | |
|---|---|---|---|---|---|---|
| Action Frequency | Do Daily | Do Daily | Do Daily | Do Weekly | Do Daily | Do Weekly |
| Nutrition Plan | Follow Plan & Schedule | Enter Observations | Evaluate & Decide | Evaluate & Decide | Make Adjustments | Make Adjustments |
| Physical Activity Plan | Follow Plan & Schedule | Enter Observations | Evaluate & Decide | Evaluate & Decide | Make Adjustments | Make Adjustments |
| Planned Items | Take Action | Enter Observations | Evaluate & Decide | Evaluate & Decide | Make Adjustments | Make Adjustments |
| Pushbacks | Manage | Enter Observations | Evaluate & Decide | Evaluate & Decide | Make Adjustments | Make Adjustments |
| Results | Accomplish | Enter Observations | Evaluate & Decide | Evaluate & Decide | Make Adjustments | Make Adjustments |

Follow-Through Items

If you are able to follow through, you should get to the destination you are committed to arrive at, and for which you have prepared well to travel. You should now have everything you need.

You are now down to start forging ahead-We wish you the BEST of luck!

# Forge

### Step 1 - Set up and Integration

In this step, you will review your weekly master schedule and complete a set of checklists we are providing to help you ensure you take the key one-time set up actions, and you complete the critical enabling activities on a weekly basis.

### Schedule Review

Open your master schedule and go over the tasks you should complete today. Continue to check your schedule as often as necessary to stay on track with your planned activities throughout the day.

The next step is to review the following checklist.

### Key Action Checklist

The number one priority should be to ensure you complete the one-time setup tasks early on. Use the checklists in the following pages to keep track of their completion.

If you prefer larger copies, you may download them from www.fitnessprotocols.com/book/forms.pdf.

One-time Task Checklists

1. Set up your fitness capabilities.

| Done | Capability Setup Checklist |
|------|----------------------------|
| | Professional advice or support |
| | Memberships to sites or fitness clubs |
| | Clothing and fitness apparel |
| | Food and drinks |
| | Food preparation and storage items |
| | Fitness equipment and gear |
| | Learning material and references |

2. Set up your environment.

| Done | Supportive Environment Setup Checklist |
|------|----------------------------------------|
| | Organize and clean your environments |
| | Eliminate bad food and drinks from your environments |
| | Display commitment certificate prominently |
| | Verify you have enough of food items on your schedule available |
| | Verify you have all the necessary food preparation items available |

3. Organize and clean up your environments.

| Done | Space Clean Sheet Cleanup Checklist |
|------|-------------------------------------|
| | Empty out everything |
| | Sort out food and drinks per the good/bad recommendations |
| | Throw or giveaway, or set aside the items that do not fit your plans |
| | Inventory all cooking accessories and equipment |
| | Cleanup spaces (food storage, refrigerator, etc.) |
| | Organize the items in some logical order back in the empty clean space |

Weekly Recurring Task Checklists

1. Ensure completion of the critical weekly enabling activities.

| Done | Weekly Enabling Routine Checklist |
|------|-----------------------------------|
| | Maintain your environments |
| | Plan and schedule the next week |
| | Do food shopping |
| | Prepare and precook food for next week |
| | Review progress and making adjustments |

2. Ensure you are maintaining supportive environments when necessary.

| Done | Supportive Environment Setup Checklist |
|---|---|
|  | Organize and clean your environments |
|  | Eliminate bad food and drinks from your environments |
|  | Display commitment certificate prominently |
|  | Verify you have enough of food items on your schedule available |
|  | Verify you have all the necessary food preparation items available |

## Step 2 - Lifestyle Plan

In this step, you will review any open action items you identified in the preparation stage (see page 181). The plan was based on your determination of possible challenges you were to encounter in your lifestyle that would limit your ability to improve your fitness. If you selected none you may skip this section. Moreover, you may choose to create a new action plan at this time. If so, you may do that in the tweaking section.

## Adjustment Steps Review

Open your master schedule to capture and go over any adjustment steps you devised. If you have not done so yet, you should transfer these action items into your master schedule to help you remember them and track any necessary action.

## Step 3 - Nutritional Plan

In this step, you will review your daily food intake plan to ensure you are following it.

Nutrition Plan Review

Refer to your plan to review and follow it.

Step 4 - Physical Activity Plan

In this step, you will review your daily physical activity plan to ensure you follow it.

Activity Plan Review

Refer to your plan to review and follow it.

Step 5 - Shopping List

In this step, you will create your weekly shopping list based on the table on page 185 and according to your daily calories number.

Use the forms on Appendix B to complete your shopping list. You may want to make copies of the form before you start.

If you prefer a larger copy, you may download it from www.fitnessprotocols.com/book/forms.pdf.

## Observe

Step 1 – Daily Observations

Nutritional Intake Observations

In this step, you will capture your daily nutritional intake observations. We will capture and summarize the information you enter here during the daily and weekly appraisal steps.

Use the form on the following page to capture your daily observations. You may want to make copies of the form before you start. You will need a copy for each meal for each day of the week.

If you prefer a larger copy, you may download it from www.fitnessprotocols.com/book/forms.pdf.

# Daily Food Intake Pattern

| | Breakfast | Morning Snack | Lunch | Afternoon Snack | Dinner | Evening Snack 1 | Evening Snack 2 |
|---|---|---|---|---|---|---|---|
| | Monday | Tuesday | Wednesday | Thursday | Friday | Saturday | Sunday |

**Food Categories**

- Cups of Veggies
- Cups of Fruit
- Tbs. of Oil
- Eq. Oz. of Protein
- Eq. Oz. of Grains
- Glasses of Water

**Food Amount**

**Meal Details**

- Meal Time
- Meal Location
- Meal Cost
- Meal Duration
- Meal Mood

**Meal Data**

Physical Activity Observations

In this step, you will capture your daily physical activity observations. We will capture and summarize the information you enter here during the daily and weekly appraisal steps.

Use the form on the following page to capture your daily observations. You may want to make copies of the form before you start. You need one copy of the form for every one of the four physical activity areas.

If you prefer a larger copy, you may download it from www.fitnessprotocols.com/book/forms.pdf.

**Daily Physical Activity Pattern**

Tabs: Regular | Cardio | Strength | Flexibility

| Day of Week | Mon | Tue | Web | Thu | Fri | Sat | Sun |
|---|---|---|---|---|---|---|---|
| Distance Covered | | | | | | | |
| Number of Steps | | | | | | | |
| Number of Reps | | | | | | | |
| Number of Sets | | | | | | | |
| Activity Intensity | | | | | | | |
| Activity Duration | | | | | | | |
| Time of Day | | | | | | | |
| Activity Location | | | | | | | |

General Observations

In this step, you will capture your daily general observations regarding follow-through, pushbacks, and the results you are getting. We will capture and summarize the information you enter here during the daily and weekly appraisal steps.

Use the form on Appendix C to capture your daily observations. You may want to make copies of the form before you start.

If you prefer a larger copy, you may download it from www.fitnessprotocols.com/book/forms.pdf.

## Appraise

Step 1 – Daily Appraisal

Here you should take a few minutes to appraise your day. If you do this right after you complete logging your observations for the day it should be fast and easy.

Use the form on the following page to get started appraising your day. You may want to make copies of the form before you start.

If you prefer a larger copy, you may download it from www.fitnessprotocols.com/book/forms.pdf.

## Daily Appraisal Process

| Appraisal Items | Appraisal Questions | YES | NO |
|---|---|---|---|
| Nutrition Plan | Does my plan need any adjustments? | | |
| | Does my schedule need any adjustments? | | |
| Physical Activity Plan | Does my plan need any adjustments? | | |
| | Does my schedule need any adjustment? | | |
| Planned Items | Are there any key pending actions I should to take soon? | | |
| Pushbacks | Is there anything I need to do to better manage a current or future condition? | | |
| | Is there anything I need to do to better manage a current or future situation? | | |
| | Is there anything I need to do to better manage my moods? | | |
| | Is there anything I need to do to better manage my habits? | | |
| | Is there anything I need to do to maintain, sustain, or increase my level of commitment? | | |
| Results | Is there anything I should do to improve my sleep? | | |
| | Is there anything I should do to reduce any old habit's pushback force? | | |
| | Is there anything I should do to help me lose weight per plan? | | |
| | Is there anything I should do to help me have more energy? | | |
| | Is there anything I should do to help me become more flexible? | | |
| | Is there anything I should do to help me have more strength? | | |

Weekly Appraisal

The first step you need to complete is to review the daily observations you made this past week.

Spend a little time going over the information you have captured during the week. Now that you have a better sense of what transpired this past week you can better appraise your progress. If your appraisal shows you are doing well, accept our congratulations, and please keep doing what you are doing.

However, if your appraisal shows some areas need improvement, consider one or all of the following questions:

- How can you improve your follow-through?
- How can you reduce the force of your top pushbacks?
- How can you become more consistent?

Use the form on the following page to capture any action items you would like to take to adjust your approach for the following week. You may want to make copies of the form before you start.

If you prefer a larger copy, you may download it from www.fitnessprotocols.com/book/forms.pdf.

## Progress Appraisal and Tweaking

| Adjustment Categories | Lifestyle Adjustments | Nutrition Adjustments | Physical Activity Adjustments |
|---|---|---|---|
| Eliminate, get rid of, throw away, stop doing, etc. | | | |
| Add, get, buy, start doing, etc. | | | |
| Reduce, minimize, avoid, do less, etc. | | | |
| Increase, accelerate, maximize, do more of, etc. | | | |

# Tweak

### Step 1 – Daily Tweaks

In this step, you will review the results of your daily appraisal step to make any necessary tweaks to your plans or schedules.

Use the form on the following page to capture your action items. Make copies of the form before you start.

If you prefer a larger copy, you may download it from www.fitnessprotocols.com/book/forms.pdf.

## Progress Appraisal and Tweaking

| Adjustment Categories | Lifestyle Adjustments | Nutrition Adjustments | Physical Activity Adjustments |
|---|---|---|---|
| Eliminate, get rid of, throw away, stop doing, etc. | | | |
| Add, get, buy, start doing, etc. | | | |
| Reduce, minimize, avoid, do less, etc. | | | |
| Increase, accelerate, maximize, do more of, etc. | | | |

Step 2 – Weekly Tweaks

In this step, you will review the results of your weekly appraisal step to make any necessary tweaks to your plans or schedules.

Once completed, make sure to capture the changes on your weekly food intake form for the following week.

Step 3 – Food Intake Plan Tweaking

In this step, you will make any changes you need to make to your food intake plan for the following week. Once completed, make sure to capture the changes on your weekly food intake form for the following week.

Step 4 – Physical Activity Plan Tweaking

In this step, you will make any changes you need to make to your physical activity plan for the following week.

Step 5 – Schedule Tweaking

In this step, you will make any changes you need to make to your master weekly schedule for the following week.

Step 6 - Shopping List Tweaking

In this step, you will make any changes you need to make to your weekly shopping list.

# Maintenance

This protocol will help you maintain the fitness improvement you have accomplished.

Fitness Maintenance

Fitness Maintenance is the fourth and final stage in the Fitness Protocol process as shown in the figure below.

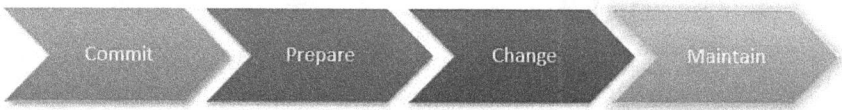

You have spent a lot of time and done a lot of work in order to get to this critical junction. Ideally, you have done so by following our protocols. Consequently, you should have accomplished the following:

- Developed a strong sense of commitment.
- Learned the basics of the mind and body.
- Set improvement targets and devised plans to help you achieve them.
- Changed your lifestyle and habits.
- Reached your improvement target.

By now, you should have reached a point where the benefits of improved fitness far outweigh the effort, as the figure below illustrates.

You should look and feel much better! Moreover, you should have more energy, strength, flexibility, and endurance. You should now be much better able to accomplish the things you want out of life. If such is the case for you, your chances of maintaining your improvement should be greatly enhanced.

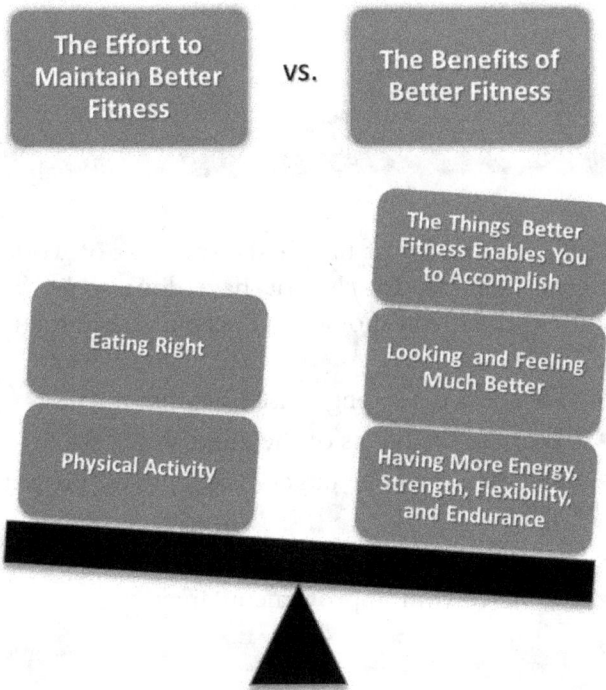

Nonetheless, a few challenges may remain. Statistics show many who reach this point are unable to maintain their accomplished improvement for an extended period.

However, the Fitness Protocols™ approach is designed to enhance your ability to maintain your fitness improvement.

As illustrated by the following figure, the "House of Fitness Maintenance" is built on a foundation of sustainable commitment, effective preparation, and life-style and habits change.

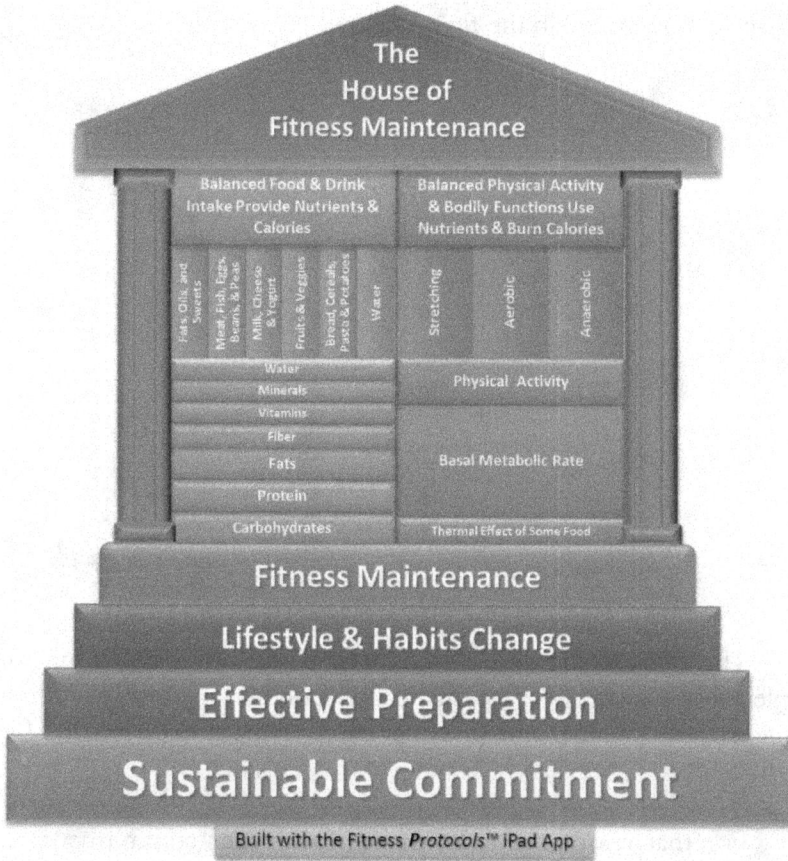

The
House of
Fitness Maintenance

Balanced Food & Drink Intake Provide Nutrients & Calories

Balanced Physical Activity & Bodily Functions Use Nutrients & Burn Calories

Fats, Oils, and Sweets | Meat, Fish, Eggs, Beans, & Peas | Milk, Cheese & Yogurt | Fruit & Veggies | Bread, Cereals, Pasta & Potatoes | Water

Stretching | Aerobic | Anaerobic

Water
Minerals
Vitamins
Fiber
Fats
Protein
Carbohydrates

Physical Activity

Basal Metabolic Rate

Thermal Effect of Some Food

Fitness Maintenance

Lifestyle & Habits Change

Effective Preparation

Sustainable Commitment

Built with the Fitness *Protocols*™ iPad App

Beating the odds will depend on how well your foundation was built, and on how well you are able to maintain energy balance moving forward. In order to remain fit, the calories from the food and drinks you consume must equal those used by daily physical activity and bodily functions.

## Maintenance Strategy

Maintaining your fitness level will require an ongoing effort to manage the dynamic tension between your commitment and the pushbacks as described in the figure below.

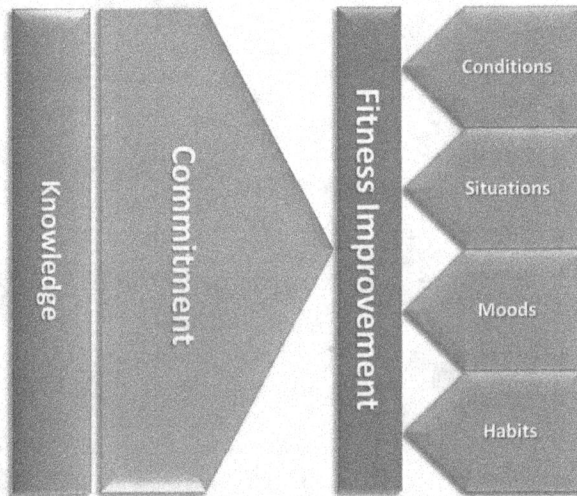

This tension should lessen as time passes. Even so, it may never completely go away because in reality, conditions change, situations emerge, moods change, and (old) habits creep back occasionally. Life is very dynamic.

For that reason, you should reinforce your commitment on an ongoing basis. Whenever you feel it starts to falter, remind yourself of the reasons you did it in the first place, and think of the benefits you are getting, and of the tremendous effort it took to get them.

However, reinforcing commitment may not be enough. Therefore, try not to abandon the enabling activities that led you to accomplish your improvement:

- Plan and schedule the upcoming week.
- Shop, prepare, and precook food per your food intake plan.
- Have the right food available at the right time.
- Observe, assess progress, and tweak your plans if necessary.
- Manage and control your key environments.
- Take time to do your physical activities.
- Come hell or high water; eat on a schedule and often.

Failure to accomplish these activities might jeopardize fitness maintenance. As you may have uncovered already, the "secret" is to allocate time for them every week! Keep making this time a top priority! This is one of the most critical habits to keep reinforcing until it is well formed.

Another critical fitness maintenance aspect is monitoring your weight. Keep getting on that scale every morning! It is the fastest way to know you are getting in trouble! Weight will fluctuate a few pounds up and down. However, it needs to remain within a decent range.

**NOTE: When you go five pounds or so over your "Maximum Ideal Weight Target," alarms should start ringing. At that point, you need to take a close look at what has changed. You need to quickly figure out what needs to be adjusted, or you will get in trouble sooner rather than later. Weight creeps on and one day you will be back where you were. Please be cognizant of that.**

Lessons Learned

We benchmarked participants in the National Weight Control Registry (NWCR) in order to validate and reinforce some of the critical success factors for fitness maintenance.

Participants in the Registry include people who have lost weight and maintained most of their weight loss for an average of five and a half years. We derived the following lessons learned from a review of the available abstracts of a number of research studies conducted using participant-provided information:

- It seems that fitness improvement can lead to improvements in energy, mobility, mood, self-confidence, and physical health.

- It seems that most participants used both diet and exercise to lose weight.

- It seems that improved fitness can reduce stress and depression in some instances.

- It seems that several years of successful weight loss maintenance increases the probability of future weight (loss) maintenance.

- It seems that weight regain can be caused in part by failure to maintain changes made during fitness improvement stage.

- It seems that weight loss maintainers use more behavioral strategies to control their weight than others do.

- It seems that dieting consistency can predict subsequent long-term weight (loss) maintenance.

- It seems that successful long-term weight loss maintainers (weight loss maintained over five years) share the following common strategies:

  o Eating a diet low in fat.
  o Frequent self-monitoring of body weight and food intake.
  o High levels of regular physical activity.

- It seems that weight loss maintenance can get easier over time.

- It seems that the chances of longer-term success greatly increase after weight loss has been maintained over two years.

- It seems that the initial sense of the effort of some of the tasks involved shifts to one of pleasure over time, further reinforcing maintenance.

If you wish to get additional details, please visit the NWCR Web site. Recruitment for the Registry is ongoing. You may join if you are at least eighteen years old and you have maintained at least a thirty-pound weight loss for one year or longer.

## Techniques, Tools, and Tricks

Following you will find a number of ideas you can use to help you with the maintenance. We recommend you scan through them so that you know what is available in case you may need to use them.

### Deep Observer

This tool can be useful for digging deep into the fitness dynamic.

A question can be a powerful tool to help us explore things. Asking them forces our attention on important aspects that might affect our effort and or results.

Follow-Through Exploration Questions

- Did you follow your food intake plan today?
- Did you follow your food intake schedule today?
- Did you follow your physical activity plan today?
- Did you follow your physical activity schedule today?
- Did you complete other plans today?

Pushbacks Exploration Questions

About Conditions

- How did your fitness level affect your plans today?
- How did your hunger level affect your plans today?
- How did your health condition affect your plans today?
- How did your comfort level affect your plans today?

About Situations

- How did occasions affect your plans today?
- How did your locations affect your plans today?
- How did available choices affect your plans today?
- How did people affect your plans today?

## About Moods

- How did your habitual thinking affect your plans today?
- How did your unmet needs affect your plans today?
- How did your circumstances affect your plans today?
- How did food or medications affect your mood today?

## About Habits

- How did your nutritional habits affect your plans today?
- How did your thinking habits affect your plans today?
- How did your physical activity habits affect you plans today?
- How did your cognitive capacities affect your plans today?
- How did any other habits affect your plans today?

## About Commitment

- How did your level of commitment affect your plans today
- How would you rate your level of commitment today?
- How did temptations affect your plans today?
- How much are the things you do not want still driving you?
- How much are the things you want badly still driving you?

Results Exploration Questions

- Did your weight change today?
- How much are old habits still pushing back?
- How well did you sleep last night?
- Is your energy level improving?
- Is your physical strength increasing?
- Are you becoming more flexible?

## Root Digger

This tool can be useful for exploring energy imbalance issues.

There is a reason or two for everything. The better we understand the reason(s), the more effective and efficient we can be at addressing the challenges we face.

Possible reasons why you have not been eating right:

- Better food is not easily available.
- Eating better is not been very convenient.
- You reverted to past eating habits or traditions.
- Eating better has become less important.
- You are back to eating food you enjoy eating.
- You cannot afford better food.
- You do not have time to eat better.

Possible reasons why you have not been as active as you should:

- Being active is not convenient.
- You reverted to past inactive habits.
- Being more active has become less important.
- You cannot afford to be active.
- A physical or health condition is preventing or limiting activity.
- You do not have enough time to be active.
- You dislike doing physical activity.

## Consequencer

This tool can be helpful for exploring the consequences of reverting to the old ways or not.

Sometimes understanding the consequences of alternatives can help redirect our effort once we realize the implication of each alternative. This evaluation can help us refocus our effort accordingly.

Use the form on the following page to capture your results. You may want to make copies of the form before you start.

If you prefer a larger copy, you may download it from www.fitnessprotocols.com/book/forms.pdf.

## What happens If...

| | | To You | To your health | To your Relationships | To your wealth |
|---|---|---|---|---|---|
| ...you revert back to your old fitness level? | 1 | | | | |
| | 2 | | | | |
| | 3 | | | | |
| ...you are able to remain fit | 1 | | | | |
| | 2 | | | | |
| | 3 | | | | |

Bias Explorer

This tool can be helpful for exploring some of the common thinking biases affecting human judgment.

Biases emerge as an easy way to cope with the sometime difficult process of making decisions. We have to make so many decisions so often that it can be overwhelming. The "lazy" brain facilitates this by enabling us to bypass the difficult process substituting thoughts for facts or reality. Understanding what biases may be affecting our judgment can help us rethink our views.

- Avoiding options for which missing information makes the probability seem unknown.
- Relying too heavily on a single piece of information or past experience when making decisions.
- Neglecting relevant data when discerning correlations or associations.
- Estimating what is more likely by what is more available in recent memory.
- Supposing a relationship between a certain type of action and an effect.
- Neglecting known odds when reevaluating odds in light of weak evidence.
- Being over-optimistic about the outcome of planned actions.
- Ignoring an obvious negative situation.
- Overestimating the probability of good things happening to them.
- Perceiving vague images or sounds as real, significant, or important.
- Expecting extreme performance to continue.
- Perceiving something to be true if beliefs demand it to be true.

## Courage Builder

This tool can be helpful for mustering courage to say NO to people and things that detract us from our fitness effort.

Whenever you are confronted with the need to say NO!, review the top reasons why you committed to improve your fitness on pages 67 and 69.

## Excuser

This tool can be helpful for evaluating whether your effort is affected by legitimate reasons or just common excuses.

Excuse making is in our human DNA. However, excuses can become problematic when they interfere with important endeavors in our life. Occasionally we need to check to make sure they do not become an issue.

Just go over the list of classic excuses people use. Simply keep your ears open for any bells ringing while you do.

- I did not have (enough) time (The NUMBER 1 excuse!)
- I ran out of...
- I forgot...
- I did not have...
- I was in a bad mood
- I was not in the mood
- I was stressed out
- I was hungry
- I could not say NO!
- I did not feel like it
- I did not have another/better option
- I had something come up

If any of these rang a bell, consider the following questions: What might the real reason behind it be? Dig a little.

Cognitive Workarounds

This tool can be helpful for identifying approaches to help overcome weak cognitive capacities.

Cognitive capabilities are the well-formed habits that can have a significant impact on follow-through we covered in the change section.

Following are suggested approaches you can consider to help you overcome issues caused by one or more of your weakest capacities.

- Emotional Control: Avoid situations that can trigger strong emotions. Start by keeping track of words, situations, and people who tend to trigger these types of emotions and devise ways to avoid them, at least for a while. If you wish to get deeper into it, you can explore the meaning you are assigning to what you see or hear to determine if it really is worth it.

- Task Initiation: Get help from technology or people. Set up reminders, alarms, etc. on your phone, computer, PDA, etc. On the other hand, have family or friends e-mail, text, call, tweet you, etc. to remind you of an action you need to take. If you can, delegate some of the tasks to others.

- Planning/Prioritization: Also, get help from technology or people. We have provided quite a planning capability in this app. However, you need to use it. Sitting down with others who may be better at this task is also a good strategy.

- Organization: Get help from others. Get help from the most organized person you know to get your environment ready. Bring the person back occasionally to help you ensure you do not lose organization. You can also hire a professional organizer to help you create and then follow a system. You can readily find these types of folks on the Web.

- Time Management: Here is another area where you can get help from technology or people. Set up reminders, alarms, etc. on your phone, computer, PDA, etc. On the other hand, have family or friends e-mail, text, call, tweet you, etc. to remind you of tasks you need to complete.

- Goal-Directed Persistence: Here you need to rely on the commitment you made. You need to keep it in front of you and refresh yourself on the commitment process you followed at the beginning. Continue to remember why you want to improve your fitness. The things you want to get away from and those you wish to gain from being fit. That is the best source of energy you can find to get you back in the game. We all have moments of doubt. We all have bad days. The key to keep us persevering is the reason why we started this in the first place.

- Flexibility: The reality is that the plans you devised will most likely change along the way. That is why we have included a tweaking step as part of the process. Eventually, and sooner than you may think, things will become stable and your need to be flexible will be less. When you find yourself struggling with change, consider exploring the underlying reason why it is so hard. Ask yourself what can happen, if you do and what can happen if you do not. That may help you flex a little.

- Metacognition: If you determine you have a hard time discerning how you are doing, consider getting feedback from others with whom you developed a strong rapport and trust. Ask them to keep an eye on you and to point out specific behaviors that may be detrimental to your effort. This action may require courage to listen and act on the feedback. However, it may be necessary.

- Stress Tolerance: Avoid conditions and situations that can trigger stress. Keep track of things causing you the most stress and do all you can to avoid them. If you wish to get deeper into it, categorize those things to determine those under your control and those outside of it. Once you have time separated, you should consider not allowing things outside your control to bother you as much. Consider and reframe what they mean to you. For the ones that you control, develop a way to address them to reduce their potential effect on you.

<u>Visualizer</u>

This tool can be helpful for building motivation and commitment.

Nothing is more powerful than our imagination. Athletes and many other successful individuals use their imagination to help them visualize success. They see themselves winning. They see themselves executing a difficult routine. Using our powerful imagination to see ourselves in the future produces great energy that we can harness to produce motivational energy. More importantly, we can use it repeatedly to remind us how we would feel once we accomplish a goal. Alternatively, if works better for you, how you would feel if you do not accomplish it.

Simply grab a piece of paper and a writing instrument and spend a few minutes composing a short imaginary news clip about how you successfully accomplished your goal and the impact it had on you and others you care most about. It is a cool experience to do this and can be helpful in reigniting your motivation and commitment if it ever fades. Just imagine how you would feel if you read that about you. Imagine how others important to you would feel. How proud would you feel? How proud would they feel? Imagine that! How does it feel?

## Do

This tool can be helpful for nudging us to take action when we do not quite feel like it.

The tool uses adaptation of strategies from the book Following Through written by Steve Levinson, PhD, and Peter Greider, M.Ed.

Spotlight - The idea is to use cues and your imagination to keep the intention or goal in mind. Posted notes with the goal on them is one way to use cues. Using the PC screen saver to repeat a mantra is another. Remind yourself of the benefits of accomplishing and the hazards of not accomplishing and use your imagination to think how you would feel one way or the other.

Block - The idea is to take an easy step today that makes it much more likely, that you will do the right thing tomorrow. Hiding or giving away the (bad) food you do not want to eat when you get hungry (out of sight, out of mind). Getting rid of clothing as you reduce weight requires you spend money if you were to gain weight back. The following metaphors offer great examples of what this strategy means:

- Locking all the exits
- Burning all the boats
- Burning all the bridges

Reasons - Great reasons provide motivational energy that helps us accomplish things and overcome temptations and obstacles in the way of accomplishing. When you have and keep remembering these reasons, they provide the power to act. Emotional energy is the key to success. You must feel the power of these reasons. They must be very important to you and not anyone else! Many successful people who become wealthy were energized by trying to prove someone wrong-someone who told them that they would not amount to anything because they did not do well in school, for example. Reasons are POWERFUL energizers of accomplishment!

Get the Horse to Water - Here the point is to get you going. When you do not feel like running, simply start walking. Ten minutes later, you may find yourself running and even enjoying every minute of it! Therefore, whenever you do not feel like it, just start with the easy part of the task, and you will be amazed what can happen after.

You may find additional useful strategies in the Follow Through book.

## Benefit Staking

This tool can be helpful for making seemingly difficult tasks seem more enticing.

You can use this tool in conjunction with the strategies above when you feel less than motivated to do something. The idea is to stack several benefits of doing a task to make it seem more enticing to complete.

Indoor Cardio

You can make exercising on stationary equipment such as treadmills and bikes seem a lot more enticing by stacking the benefits and pleasures of certain activities. You can watch a movie, or TV show, read a book, or surf the Web while you exercise.

Reading makes time seem to pass very fast! Moreover, you get the benefit of enjoying what you read, learning new things, or catching up on the latest news (or gossip if you are into that kind of stuff). However, you can only read comfortably up to speeds of about 4 mph. On the other hand, you can watch a TV show or a movie at any speed and get still the benefit of making time seem to go faster.

Besides the obvious fitness benefits and those we mentioned before, a good workout can reduce stress, and can help make you sleep much better. Paradoxically, doing exercise when you feel tired can make you feel energized afterward.

So next time you do not feel like doing some walking, think of all the good things you can get out of it almost immediately.

Outdoor Cardio

You can make outdoor walking or jogging seem a lot more enticing by stacking the benefits and pleasures of certain activities. You can listen to some good tunes, radio news, talk shows, or audio books while you walk or jog. You can also benefit from breathing fresh air, getting vitamin D from the sun, and enjoying nature if you have safe access to a nice park or other trails. Being outdoors also enables you to meet people who enjoy similar activities. Once again, these benefits stack up and can make tasks like these seem a lot more enticing.

There are a lot more benefits to these activities that you first think. Just think about them and stack them up to make them more enticing to you. You will be amazed!

Failure Planner

Anticipating and planning for failure can be an effective strategy to mitigate its effect. When you do not plan to fail, you can get easily discouraged. Unfortunately, discouragement is one of the most common reasons why some fitness efforts end abruptly.

To prepare better, you need to spend time identifying ways in which things can go wrong. Here are some common failures that can get you discouraged:

- Failure to lose weight
- Failure to stick to the food plan
- Failure to stick to the physical activity plan
- Failure to control an old habit
- Failure to control temptations
- Failure to control your environment

Consider these and any others you can come up with and develop simple contingency plans for when they happen. It will go a long way in mitigating the discouragement that can come from unplanned failure.

# Your best is yet to come!

# Appendix A

Calorie Burning Chart by Activity and Weight for 150-170 Lbs.

| Estimates for One Hour of Physical Effort | 150 | 155 | 160 | 165 | 170 |
|---|---|---|---|---|---|
| Aerobics | 442 | 457 | 472 | 487 | 502 |
| Aerobics, high impact | 477 | 493 | 508 | 524 | 540 |
| Aerobics, low impact | 341 | 352 | 364 | 375 | 386 |
| Aerobics, step aerobics | 579 | 598 | 618 | 637 | 656 |
| Bagging grass, leaves | 272 | 281 | 291 | 300 | 309 |
| Ballroom dancing, fast | 375 | 387 | 399 | 412 | 424 |
| Ballroom dancing, slow | 204 | 211 | 218 | 225 | 231 |
| Basketball, shooting baskets | 307 | 317 | 327 | 337 | 348 |
| Canoeing, rowing, light | 204 | 211 | 218 | 225 | 231 |
| Canoeing, rowing, moderate | 477 | 493 | 508 | 524 | 540 |
| Cross country skiing, moderate | 545 | 563 | 581 | 600 | 618 |
| Cross country snow skiing, slow | 477 | 493 | 508 | 524 | 540 |
| Cycling at an average of 11 mph | 408 | 422 | 436 | 449 | 463 |
| Cycling under 10 mph | 272 | 281 | 291 | 300 | 309 |
| Downhill snow skiing, moderate | 408 | 422 | 436 | 449 | 463 |
| Fencing | 408 | 422 | 436 | 449 | 463 |
| Frisbee playing, general | 204 | 211 | 218 | 225 | 231 |
| Gardening, general | 272 | 281 | 291 | 300 | 309 |
| General cleaning | 238 | 246 | 254 | 262 | 270 |
| General housework | 238 | 246 | 254 | 262 | 270 |
| Golf, driving range | 204 | 211 | 218 | 225 | 231 |
| Golf, general | 307 | 317 | 327 | 337 | 348 |
| Golf, miniature golf | 204 | 211 | 218 | 225 | 231 |
| Golf, using power cart | 238 | 246 | 254 | 262 | 270 |
| Golf, walking and carrying clubs | 307 | 317 | 327 | 337 | 348 |
| Golf, walking and pulling clubs | 293 | 303 | 312 | 322 | 332 |
| Handball | 817 | 844 | 872 | 899 | 927 |
| Ice skating, < 9 mph | 375 | 387 | 399 | 412 | 424 |
| Ice skating, average speed | 477 | 493 | 508 | 524 | 540 |
| Ice skating, rapidly | 613 | 633 | 653 | 674 | 694 |
| Jazzercise | 408 | 422 | 436 | 449 | 463 |
| Jumping rope, moderate | 681 | 704 | 726 | 749 | 772 |
| Jumping rope, slow | 545 | 563 | 581 | 600 | 618 |
| Kayaking | 341 | 352 | 364 | 375 | 386 |
| Mild stretching | 170 | 176 | 181 | 187 | 193 |
| Mowing lawn, walk, power mower | 375 | 387 | 399 | 412 | 424 |
| Playing basketball, non game | 408 | 422 | 436 | 449 | 463 |
| Playing paddleball | 408 | 422 | 436 | 449 | 463 |
| Playing racquetball | 477 | 493 | 508 | 524 | 540 |

All estimates are based on data from the American College of Sports Medicine.

# Calorie Burning Chart by Activity and Weight for 150-170 Lbs.

| Estimates for One Hour of Physical Effort | 150 | 155 | 160 | 165 | 170 |
|---|---|---|---|---|---|
| Playing soccer | 477 | 493 | 508 | 524 | 540 |
| Playing tennis | 477 | 493 | 508 | 524 | 540 |
| Playing volleyball | 204 | 211 | 218 | 225 | 231 |
| Raking lawn | 293 | 303 | 312 | 322 | 332 |
| Rock climbing, rappelling | 545 | 563 | 581 | 600 | 618 |
| Roller blading, in-line skating | 817 | 844 | 872 | 899 | 927 |
| Roller skating | 477 | 493 | 508 | 524 | 540 |
| Rowing machine, light | 238 | 246 | 254 | 262 | 270 |
| Rowing machine, moderate | 477 | 493 | 508 | 524 | 540 |
| Rowing machine, vigorous | 579 | 598 | 618 | 637 | 656 |
| Running, 5 mph (12 minute mile) | 545 | 563 | 581 | 600 | 618 |
| Running, 6 mph (10 min mile) | 681 | 704 | 726 | 749 | 772 |
| Running, 7 mph (8.5 min mile) | 783 | 809 | 836 | 862 | 888 |
| Shoveling snow by hand | 408 | 422 | 436 | 449 | 463 |
| Snow skiing, downhill skiing, light | 341 | 352 | 364 | 375 | 386 |
| Squash | 817 | 844 | 872 | 899 | 927 |
| Stair machine | 613 | 633 | 653 | 674 | 694 |
| Standing, playing with children, light | 191 | 197 | 204 | 210 | 216 |
| Stationary cycling, light | 375 | 387 | 399 | 412 | 424 |
| Stationary cycling, moderate | 477 | 493 | 508 | 524 | 540 |
| Stationary cycling, very light | 204 | 211 | 218 | 225 | 231 |
| Stretching, hatha yoga | 272 | 281 | 291 | 300 | 309 |
| Swimming laps, freestyle, fast | 681 | 704 | 726 | 749 | 772 |
| Swimming laps, freestyle, slow | 477 | 493 | 508 | 524 | 540 |
| Swimming leisurely, not laps | 408 | 422 | 436 | 449 | 463 |
| Swimming, treading water, moderate | 272 | 281 | 291 | 300 | 309 |
| Table tennis, ping pong | 272 | 281 | 291 | 300 | 309 |
| Trampoline | 238 | 246 | 254 | 262 | 270 |
| Volleyball, beach | 545 | 563 | 581 | 600 | 618 |
| Walk/run, playing with children, moderate | 272 | 281 | 291 | 300 | 309 |
| Walk/run, playing with children, vigorous | 341 | 352 | 364 | 375 | 386 |
| Walking 3.0 mph, moderate | 225 | 232 | 240 | 248 | 255 |
| Walking 3.5 mph, brisk pace | 258 | 267 | 276 | 285 | 294 |
| Walking 3.5 mph, uphill | 408 | 422 | 436 | 449 | 463 |
| Walking 4.0 mph, very brisk | 341 | 352 | 364 | 375 | 386 |
| Walking, snow blower | 238 | 246 | 254 | 262 | 270 |
| Water aerobics | 272 | 281 | 291 | 300 | 309 |
| Weeding, cultivating garden | 307 | 317 | 327 | 337 | 348 |
| Weight lifting, light workout | 204 | 211 | 218 | 225 | 231 |

All estimates are based on data from the American College of Sports Medicine.

# Calorie Burning Chart by Activity and Weight for 175-200 Lbs.

| Estimates for One Hour of Physical Effort | 175 | 180 | 185 | 190 | 195 | 200 |
|---|---|---|---|---|---|---|
| Aerobics | 516 | 531 | 546 | 561 | 575 | 590 |
| Aerobics, high impact | 556 | 572 | 587 | 603 | 619 | 635 |
| Aerobics, low impact | 398 | 409 | 420 | 431 | 442 | 454 |
| Aerobics, step aerobics | 676 | 695 | 714 | 733 | 752 | 772 |
| Bagging grass, leaves | 318 | 327 | 336 | 345 | 354 | 363 |
| Ballroom dancing, fast | 437 | 449 | 462 | 475 | 487 | 500 |
| Ballroom dancing, slow | 238 | 245 | 252 | 259 | 265 | 272 |
| Basketball, shooting baskets | 358 | 368 | 378 | 388 | 399 | 409 |
| Canoeing, rowing, light | 238 | 245 | 252 | 259 | 265 | 272 |
| Canoeing, rowing, moderate | 556 | 572 | 587 | 603 | 619 | 635 |
| Cross country skiing, moderate | 636 | 654 | 672 | 690 | 709 | 727 |
| Cross country snow skiing, slow | 556 | 572 | 587 | 603 | 619 | 635 |
| Cycling at an average of 11 mph | 476 | 490 | 504 | 517 | 531 | 544 |
| Cycling under 10 mph | 318 | 327 | 336 | 345 | 354 | 363 |
| Downhill snow skiing, moderate | 476 | 490 | 504 | 517 | 531 | 544 |
| Fencing | 476 | 490 | 504 | 517 | 531 | 544 |
| Frisbee playing, general | 238 | 245 | 252 | 259 | 265 | 272 |
| Gardening, general | 318 | 327 | 336 | 345 | 354 | 363 |
| General cleaning | 278 | 286 | 294 | 302 | 310 | 318 |
| General housework | 278 | 286 | 294 | 302 | 310 | 318 |
| Golf, driving range | 238 | 245 | 252 | 259 | 265 | 272 |
| Golf, general | 358 | 368 | 378 | 388 | 399 | 409 |
| Golf, miniature golf | 238 | 245 | 252 | 259 | 265 | 272 |
| Golf, using power cart | 278 | 286 | 294 | 302 | 310 | 318 |
| Golf, walking and carrying clubs | 358 | 368 | 378 | 388 | 399 | 409 |
| Golf, walking and pulling clubs | 341 | 351 | 361 | 371 | 380 | 390 |
| Handball | 954 | 981 | 1008 | 1035 | 1063 | 1090 |
| Ice skating, < 9 mph | 437 | 449 | 462 | 475 | 487 | 500 |
| Ice skating, average speed | 556 | 572 | 587 | 603 | 619 | 635 |
| Ice skating, rapidly | 715 | 735 | 756 | 777 | 797 | 818 |
| Jazzercise | 476 | 490 | 504 | 517 | 531 | 544 |
| Jumping rope, moderate | 794 | 817 | 840 | 863 | 886 | 908 |
| Jumping rope, slow | 636 | 654 | 672 | 690 | 709 | 727 |
| Kayaking | 398 | 409 | 420 | 431 | 442 | 454 |
| Mild stretching | 198 | 204 | 210 | 216 | 222 | 227 |
| Mowing lawn, walk, power mower | 437 | 449 | 462 | 475 | 487 | 500 |
| Playing basketball, non game | 476 | 490 | 504 | 517 | 531 | 544 |
| Playing paddleball | 476 | 490 | 504 | 517 | 531 | 544 |
| Playing racquetball | 556 | 572 | 587 | 603 | 619 | 635 |

All estimates are based on data from the American College of Sports Medicine.

## Calorie Burning Chart by Activity and Weight for 175-200 Lbs.

| Estimates for One Hour of Physical Effort | 175 | 180 | 185 | 190 | 195 | 200 |
|---|---|---|---|---|---|---|
| Playing soccer | 556 | 572 | 587 | 603 | 619 | 635 |
| Playing tennis | 556 | 572 | 587 | 603 | 619 | 635 |
| Playing volleyball | 238 | 245 | 252 | 259 | 265 | 272 |
| Raking lawn | 341 | 351 | 361 | 371 | 380 | 390 |
| Rock climbing, rappelling | 636 | 654 | 672 | 690 | 709 | 727 |
| Roller blading, in-line skating | 954 | 981 | 1008 | 1035 | 1063 | 1090 |
| Roller skating | 556 | 572 | 587 | 603 | 619 | 635 |
| Rowing machine, light | 278 | 286 | 294 | 302 | 310 | 318 |
| Rowing machine, moderate | 556 | 572 | 587 | 603 | 619 | 635 |
| Rowing machine, vigorous | 676 | 695 | 714 | 733 | 752 | 772 |
| Running, 5 mph (12 minute mile) | 636 | 654 | 672 | 690 | 709 | 727 |
| Running, 6 mph (10 min mile) | 794 | 817 | 840 | 863 | 886 | 908 |
| Running, 7 mph (8.5 min mile) | 914 | 940 | 966 | 992 | 1018 | 1044 |
| Shoveling snow by hand | 476 | 490 | 504 | 517 | 531 | 544 |
| Snow skiing, downhill skiing, light | 398 | 409 | 420 | 431 | 442 | 454 |
| Squash | 954 | 981 | 1008 | 1035 | 1063 | 1090 |
| Stair machine | 715 | 735 | 756 | 777 | 797 | 818 |
| Standing, playing with children, light | 223 | 229 | 236 | 242 | 248 | 255 |
| Stationary cycling, light | 437 | 449 | 462 | 475 | 487 | 500 |
| Stationary cycling, moderate | 556 | 572 | 587 | 603 | 619 | 635 |
| Stationary cycling, very light | 238 | 245 | 252 | 259 | 265 | 272 |
| Stretching, hatha yoga | 318 | 327 | 336 | 345 | 354 | 363 |
| Swimming laps, freestyle, fast | 794 | 817 | 840 | 863 | 886 | 908 |
| Swimming laps, freestyle, slow | 556 | 572 | 587 | 603 | 619 | 635 |
| Swimming leisurely, not laps | 476 | 490 | 504 | 517 | 531 | 544 |
| Swimming, treading water, moderate | 318 | 327 | 336 | 345 | 354 | 363 |
| Table tennis, ping pong | 318 | 327 | 336 | 345 | 354 | 363 |
| Trampoline | 278 | 286 | 294 | 302 | 310 | 318 |
| Volleyball, beach | 636 | 654 | 672 | 690 | 709 | 727 |
| Walk/run, playing with children, moderate | 318 | 327 | 336 | 345 | 354 | 363 |
| Walk/run, playing with children, vigorous | 398 | 409 | 420 | 431 | 442 | 454 |
| Walking 3.0 mph, moderate | 263 | 270 | 277 | 285 | 292 | 300 |
| Walking 3.5 mph, brisk pace | 302 | 311 | 319 | 328 | 337 | 345 |
| Walking 3.5 mph, uphill | 476 | 490 | 504 | 517 | 531 | 544 |
| Walking 4.0 mph, very brisk | 398 | 409 | 420 | 431 | 442 | 454 |
| Walking, snow blower | 278 | 286 | 294 | 302 | 310 | 318 |
| Water aerobics | 318 | 327 | 336 | 345 | 354 | 363 |
| Weeding, cultivating garden | 358 | 368 | 378 | 388 | 399 | 409 |
| Weight lifting, light workout | 238 | 245 | 252 | 259 | 265 | 272 |

All estimates are based on data from the American College of Sports Medicine.

# Calorie Burning Chart by Activity and Weight for 205-225 Lbs.

| Estimates for One Hour of Physical Effort | 205 | 210 | 215 | 220 | 225 |
|---|---|---|---|---|---|
| Aerobics | 605 | 620 | 635 | 649 | 664 |
| Aerobics, high impact | 651 | 667 | 683 | 699 | 715 |
| Aerobics, low impact | 465 | 476 | 488 | 499 | 510 |
| Aerobics, step aerobics | 791 | 810 | 830 | 849 | 868 |
| Bagging grass, leaves | 372 | 381 | 390 | 399 | 408 |
| Ballroom dancing, fast | 512 | 524 | 537 | 549 | 562 |
| Ballroom dancing, slow | 279 | 286 | 293 | 299 | 306 |
| Basketball, shooting baskets | 419 | 429 | 439 | 450 | 460 |
| Canoeing, rowing, light | 279 | 286 | 293 | 299 | 306 |
| Canoeing, rowing, moderate | 651 | 667 | 683 | 699 | 715 |
| Cross country skiing, moderate | 745 | 763 | 781 | 800 | 818 |
| Cross country snow skiing, slow | 651 | 667 | 683 | 699 | 715 |
| Cycling at an average of 11 mph | 558 | 572 | 585 | 599 | 612 |
| Cycling under 10 mph | 372 | 381 | 390 | 399 | 408 |
| Downhill snow skiing, moderate | 558 | 572 | 585 | 599 | 612 |
| Fencing | 558 | 572 | 585 | 599 | 612 |
| Frisbee playing, general | 279 | 286 | 293 | 299 | 306 |
| Gardening, general | 372 | 381 | 390 | 399 | 408 |
| General cleaning | 326 | 334 | 342 | 350 | 358 |
| General housework | 326 | 334 | 342 | 350 | 358 |
| Golf, driving range | 279 | 286 | 293 | 299 | 306 |
| Golf, general | 419 | 429 | 439 | 450 | 460 |
| Golf, miniature golf | 279 | 286 | 293 | 299 | 306 |
| Golf, using power cart | 326 | 334 | 342 | 350 | 358 |
| Golf, walking and carrying clubs | 419 | 429 | 439 | 450 | 460 |
| Golf, walking and pulling clubs | 400 | 410 | 420 | 429 | 439 |
| Handball | 1117 | 1144 | 1171 | 1199 | 1226 |
| Ice skating, < 9 mph | 512 | 524 | 537 | 549 | 562 |
| Ice skating, average speed | 651 | 667 | 683 | 699 | 715 |
| Ice skating, rapidly | 838 | 858 | 879 | 899 | 920 |
| Jazzercise | 558 | 572 | 585 | 599 | 612 |
| Jumping rope, moderate | 931 | 954 | 976 | 999 | 1022 |
| Jumping rope, slow | 745 | 763 | 781 | 800 | 818 |
| Kayaking | 465 | 476 | 488 | 499 | 510 |
| Mild stretching | 233 | 239 | 244 | 250 | 256 |
| Mowing lawn, walk, power mower | 512 | 524 | 537 | 549 | 562 |
| Playing basketball, non game | 558 | 572 | 585 | 599 | 612 |
| Playing paddleball | 558 | 572 | 585 | 599 | 612 |

All estimates are based on data from the American College of Sports Medicine.

Calorie Burning Chart by Activity and Weight for 205-225 Lbs.

| Estimates for One Hour of Physical Effort | 205 | 210 | 215 | 220 | 225 |
|---|---|---|---|---|---|
| Playing racquetball | 651 | 667 | 683 | 699 | 715 |
| Playing soccer | 651 | 667 | 683 | 699 | 715 |
| Playing tennis | 651 | 667 | 683 | 699 | 715 |
| Playing volleyball | 279 | 286 | 293 | 299 | 306 |
| Raking lawn | 400 | 410 | 420 | 429 | 439 |
| Rock climbing, rappelling | 745 | 763 | 781 | 800 | 818 |
| Roller blading, in-line skating | 1117 | 1144 | 1171 | 1199 | 1226 |
| Roller skating | 651 | 667 | 683 | 699 | 715 |
| Rowing machine, light | 326 | 334 | 342 | 350 | 358 |
| Rowing machine, moderate | 651 | 667 | 683 | 699 | 715 |
| Rowing machine, vigorous | 791 | 810 | 830 | 849 | 868 |
| Running, 5 mph (12 minute mile) | 745 | 763 | 781 | 800 | 818 |
| Running, 6 mph (10 min mile) | 931 | 954 | 976 | 999 | 1022 |
| Running, 7 mph (8.5 min mile) | 1070 | 1096 | 1122 | 1148 | 1174 |
| Shoveling snow by hand | 558 | 572 | 585 | 599 | 612 |
| Snow skiing, downhill skiing, light | 465 | 476 | 488 | 499 | 510 |
| Squash | 1117 | 1144 | 1171 | 1199 | 1226 |
| Stair machine | 838 | 858 | 879 | 899 | 920 |
| Standing, playing with children, light | 261 | 267 | 274 | 280 | 286 |
| Stationary cycling, light | 512 | 524 | 537 | 549 | 562 |
| Stationary cycling, moderate | 651 | 667 | 683 | 699 | 715 |
| Stationary cycling, very light | 279 | 286 | 293 | 299 | 306 |
| Stretching, hatha yoga | 372 | 381 | 390 | 399 | 408 |
| Swimming laps, freestyle, fast | 931 | 954 | 976 | 999 | 1022 |
| Swimming laps, freestyle, slow | 651 | 667 | 683 | 699 | 715 |
| Swimming leisurely, not laps | 558 | 572 | 585 | 599 | 612 |
| Swimming, treading water, moderate | 372 | 381 | 390 | 399 | 408 |
| Table tennis, ping pong | 372 | 381 | 390 | 399 | 408 |
| Trampoline | 326 | 334 | 342 | 350 | 358 |
| Volleyball, beach | 745 | 763 | 781 | 800 | 818 |
| Walk/run, playing with children, moderate | 372 | 381 | 390 | 399 | 408 |
| Walk/run, playing with children, vigorous | 465 | 476 | 488 | 499 | 510 |
| Walking 3.0 mph, moderate | 307 | 314 | 322 | 329 | 337 |
| Walking 3.5 mph, brisk pace | 354 | 363 | 371 | 380 | 389 |
| Walking 3.5 mph, uphill | 558 | 572 | 585 | 599 | 612 |
| Walking 4.0 mph, very brisk | 465 | 476 | 488 | 499 | 510 |
| Walking, snow blower | 326 | 334 | 342 | 350 | 358 |
| Water aerobics | 372 | 381 | 390 | 399 | 408 |
| Weeding, cultivating garden | 419 | 429 | 439 | 450 | 460 |
| Weight lifting, light workout | 279 | 286 | 293 | 299 | 306 |

All estimates are based on data from the American College of Sports Medicine.

# Calorie Burning Chart by Activity and Weight for 230-250 Lbs.

| Estimates for One Hour of Physical Effort | 230 | 235 | 240 | 245 | 250 |
|---|---|---|---|---|---|
| Aerobics | 679 | 694 | 708 | 723 | 738 |
| Aerobics, high impact | 730 | 746 | 762 | 778 | 794 |
| Aerobics, low impact | 522 | 533 | 544 | 556 | 567 |
| Aerobics, step aerobics | 887 | 907 | 926 | 945 | 965 |
| Bagging grass, leaves | 417 | 426 | 436 | 445 | 454 |
| Ballroom dancing, fast | 574 | 587 | 599 | 612 | 624 |
| Ballroom dancing, slow | 313 | 320 | 327 | 333 | 340 |
| Basketball, shooting baskets | 470 | 480 | 491 | 501 | 511 |
| Canoeing, rowing, light | 313 | 320 | 327 | 333 | 340 |
| Canoeing, rowing, moderate | 730 | 746 | 762 | 778 | 794 |
| Cross country skiing, moderate | 836 | 854 | 872 | 890 | 909 |
| Cross country snow skiing, slow | 730 | 746 | 762 | 778 | 794 |
| Cycling at an average of 11 mph | 626 | 640 | 653 | 667 | 680 |
| Cycling under 10 mph | 417 | 426 | 436 | 445 | 454 |
| Downhill snow skiing, moderate | 626 | 640 | 653 | 667 | 680 |
| Fencing | 626 | 640 | 653 | 667 | 680 |
| Frisbee playing, general | 313 | 320 | 327 | 333 | 340 |
| Gardening, general | 417 | 426 | 436 | 445 | 454 |
| General cleaning | 366 | 374 | 382 | 390 | 398 |
| General housework | 366 | 374 | 382 | 390 | 398 |
| Golf, driving range | 313 | 320 | 327 | 333 | 340 |
| Golf, general | 470 | 480 | 491 | 501 | 511 |
| Golf, miniature golf | 313 | 320 | 327 | 333 | 340 |
| Golf, using power cart | 366 | 374 | 382 | 390 | 398 |
| Golf, walking and carrying clubs | 470 | 480 | 491 | 501 | 511 |
| Golf, walking and pulling clubs | 449 | 459 | 468 | 478 | 488 |
| Handball | 1253 | 1280 | 1308 | 1335 | 1362 |
| Ice skating, < 9 mph | 574 | 587 | 599 | 612 | 624 |
| Ice skating, average speed | 730 | 746 | 762 | 778 | 794 |
| Ice skating, rapidly | 940 | 961 | 981 | 1002 | 1022 |
| Jazzercise | 626 | 640 | 653 | 667 | 680 |
| Jumping rope, moderate | 1045 | 1067 | 1090 | 1113 | 1135 |
| Jumping rope, slow | 836 | 854 | 872 | 890 | 909 |
| Kayaking | 522 | 533 | 544 | 556 | 567 |
| Mild stretching | 261 | 267 | 273 | 278 | 284 |
| Mowing lawn, walk, power mower | 574 | 587 | 599 | 612 | 624 |
| Playing basketball, non game | 626 | 640 | 653 | 667 | 680 |
| Playing paddleball | 626 | 640 | 653 | 667 | 680 |

All estimates are based on data from the American College of Sports Medicine.

# Calorie Burning Chart by Activity and Weight for 230-250 Lbs.

| Estimates for One Hour of Physical Effort | 230 | 235 | 240 | 245 | 250 |
|---|---|---|---|---|---|
| Playing racquetball | 730 | 746 | 762 | 778 | 794 |
| Playing soccer | 730 | 746 | 762 | 778 | 794 |
| Playing tennis | 730 | 746 | 762 | 778 | 794 |
| Playing volleyball | 313 | 320 | 327 | 333 | 340 |
| Raking lawn | 449 | 459 | 468 | 478 | 488 |
| Rock climbing, rappelling | 836 | 854 | 872 | 890 | 909 |
| Roller blading, in-line skating | 1253 | 1280 | 1308 | 1335 | 1362 |
| Roller skating | 730 | 746 | 762 | 778 | 794 |
| Rowing machine, light | 366 | 374 | 382 | 390 | 398 |
| Rowing machine, moderate | 730 | 746 | 762 | 778 | 794 |
| Rowing machine, vigorous | 887 | 907 | 926 | 945 | 965 |
| Running, 5 mph (12 minute mile) | 836 | 854 | 872 | 890 | 909 |
| Running, 6 mph (10 min mile) | 1045 | 1067 | 1090 | 1113 | 1135 |
| Running, 7 mph (8.5 min mile) | 1200 | 1227 | 1253 | 1279 | 1305 |
| Shoveling snow by hand | 626 | 640 | 653 | 667 | 680 |
| Snow skiing, downhill skiing, light | 522 | 533 | 544 | 556 | 567 |
| Squash | 1253 | 1280 | 1308 | 1335 | 1362 |
| Stair machine | 940 | 961 | 981 | 1002 | 1022 |
| Standing, playing with children, light | 293 | 299 | 306 | 312 | 318 |
| Stationary cycling, light | 574 | 587 | 599 | 612 | 624 |
| Stationary cycling, moderate | 730 | 746 | 762 | 778 | 794 |
| Stationary cycling, very light | 313 | 320 | 327 | 333 | 340 |
| Stretching, hatha yoga | 417 | 426 | 436 | 445 | 454 |
| Swimming laps, freestyle, fast | 1045 | 1067 | 1090 | 1113 | 1135 |
| Swimming laps, freestyle, slow | 730 | 746 | 762 | 778 | 794 |
| Swimming leisurely, not laps | 626 | 640 | 653 | 667 | 680 |
| Swimming, treading water, moderate | 417 | 426 | 436 | 445 | 454 |
| Table tennis, ping pong | 417 | 426 | 436 | 445 | 454 |
| Trampoline | 366 | 374 | 382 | 390 | 398 |
| Volleyball, beach | 836 | 854 | 872 | 890 | 909 |
| Walk/run, playing with children, moderate | 417 | 426 | 436 | 445 | 454 |
| Walk/run, playing with children, vigorous | 522 | 533 | 544 | 556 | 567 |
| Walking 3.0 mph, moderate | 344 | 352 | 359 | 367 | 374 |
| Walking 3.5 mph, brisk pace | 397 | 406 | 414 | 423 | 432 |
| Walking 3.5 mph, uphill | 626 | 640 | 653 | 667 | 680 |
| Walking 4.0 mph, very brisk | 522 | 533 | 544 | 556 | 567 |
| Walking, snow blower | 366 | 374 | 382 | 390 | 398 |
| Water aerobics | 417 | 426 | 436 | 445 | 454 |
| Weeding, cultivating garden | 470 | 480 | 491 | 501 | 511 |
| Weight lifting, light workout | 313 | 320 | 327 | 333 | 340 |

All estimates are based on data from the American College of Sports Medicine.

# Appendix B
## Shopping List Forms

### Weekly Food Shopping List

| Vegetables | Fruit | Oils | Protein | Grains | Other |
|---|---|---|---|---|---|

| Dark Green | | Orange | | Starchy | | Legumes | | Other Veggies | |
|---|---|---|---|---|---|---|---|---|---|
| Item | Qty. | Item | Qty. | Item | Qty. | Item | Qty. | Item | Qty. |
| | | | | | | | | | |
| | | | | | | | | | |
| | | | | | | | | | |
| | | | | | | | | | |
| | | | | | | | | | |
| | | | | | | | | | |
| | | | | | | | | | |
| | | | | | | | | | |
| | | | | | | | | | |
| | | | | | | | | | |
| | | | | | | | | | |
| | | | | | | | | | |
| | | | | | | | | | |

# Weekly Food Shopping List

| Vegetables | Fruit | Oils | Protein | Grains | Other |
|---|---|---|---|---|---|

| Item | Qty. |
|---|---|
|  |  |
|  |  |
|  |  |
|  |  |
|  |  |
|  |  |
|  |  |
|  |  |
|  |  |
|  |  |
|  |  |

# Weekly Food Shopping List

| Vegetables | Fruit | Oils | Protein | Grains | Other |
|---|---|---|---|---|---|

| Item | Qty. |
|---|---|
| | |
| | |
| | |
| | |
| | |
| | |
| | |
| | |
| | |
| | |
| | |

# Weekly Food Shopping List

| Vegetables | Fruit | Oils | Protein | Grains | Other |
|---|---|---|---|---|---|

| Meat and Poultry | | Fish & Seafood | | Eggs | | Dry Beans & Peas | | Nuts & Seeds | |
|---|---|---|---|---|---|---|---|---|---|
| Item | Qty. | Item | Qty. | Item | Qty. | Item | Qty. | Item | Qty. |
| | | | | | | | | | |
| | | | | | | | | | |
| | | | | | | | | | |
| | | | | | | | | | |
| | | | | | | | | | |
| | | | | | | | | | |
| | | | | | | | | | |
| | | | | | | | | | |
| | | | | | | | | | |
| | | | | | | | | | |
| | | | | | | | | | |
| | | | | | | | | | |

# Weekly Food Shopping List

| Vegetables | Fruit | Oils | Protein | Grains | Other |
|---|---|---|---|---|---|

| Bread | | Cereal | | Rice | | Pasta | | Other | |
|---|---|---|---|---|---|---|---|---|---|
| Item | Qty. | Item | Qty. | Item | Qty. | Item | Qty. | Item | Qty. |
| | | | | | | | | | |
| | | | | | | | | | |
| | | | | | | | | | |
| | | | | | | | | | |
| | | | | | | | | | |
| | | | | | | | | | |
| | | | | | | | | | |
| | | | | | | | | | |
| | | | | | | | | | |
| | | | | | | | | | |

# Weekly Food Shopping List

| Vegetables | Fruit | Oils | Protein | Grains | Other |
|---|---|---|---|---|---|

| Item | Qty. |
|---|---|
| | |
| | |
| | |
| | |
| | |
| | |
| | |
| | |
| | |
| | |
| | |

# Appendix C
## Observations Forms

| Follow-Through | Pushbacks | Results |

| Observations | | Conditions |
|---|---|---|
| How well did you follow though? | | Situations |
| **Action Items** | **Observation** | Moods |
| How much did you plan and <u>prepare</u>? | | Habits |
| How much did you follow your <u>plans</u>? | | |
| How much did you adhere to your master <u>schedule</u>? | | Commitment |

| Follow-Through | Pushbacks | Results |

| Observations | | Conditions |
|---|---|---|
| What were the strongest forces pushing back against your commitment? | | Situations |
| **Pushbacks Forces** | **Observation** | Moods |
| You <u>fitness level</u> | | Habits |
| Your <u>hunger</u> | | |
| Your <u>health condition</u> | | Commitment |
| Your <u>physical comfort</u> level | | |

| Follow-Through | Pushbacks | Results |

| Conditions |
| Situations |
| Moods |
| Habits |
| Commitment |

## Observations

What were the strongest forces pushing back against your commitment?

| Pushbacks Forces | Observation |
| --- | --- |
| Social occasions | |
| Locations/environments | |
| Available food choices | |
| People | |

---

| Follow-Through | Pushbacks | Results |

| Conditions |
| Situations |
| Moods |
| Habits |
| Commitment |

## Observations

What were the strongest forces pushing back against your commitment?

| Pushbacks Forces | Observation |
| --- | --- |
| Your habitual thinking | |
| Your unmet needs | |
| Your circumstances | |
| Your medications | |

## Observations

What were the strongest forces pushing back against your commitment?

| Pushbacks Forces | Observation |
|---|---|
| Your nutritional habits | |
| Your thinking habits | |
| Your physical activity habits | |
| Your weak cognitive capacities | |
| Other habits | |

Tabs (right side): Conditions, Situations, Moods, **Habits**, Commitment

---

## Observations

Your level of commitment

| Pushbacks Forces | Observation |
|---|---|
| Rate your level of commitment | |

Tabs (right side): Conditions, Situations, Moods, Habits, **Commitment**

| | |
|---|---|
| Follow-Through | Pushbacks | **Results** |

| Observations | |
|---|---|
| **Observations** | Conditions |
| What results were you able to accomplish? | |
| **Results Accomplished** | **Observation** |
| How much did you weight today? | |
| How much energy did you have? | |
| How well did you sleep? | |
| How much strength did you have? | |
| How much flexibility did you have? | |
| How much time did you spend feeling good? | |

Side tabs: Conditions, Situations, Moods, Habits, Commitment

# Index

Activity Balance, 133

Activity Patterns, 153

Aerobic, 137

Agility, 149

Anaerobic, 137

Appraising, 220

approach, 1, 2, 3, 4, 5, 6, 50, 53, 85, 86, 94, 95, 96, 97, 100, 101, 104, 114, 120, 134, 135, 139, 143, 144, 149, 158, 162, 165, 171, 174, 175, 182, 188, 193, 194, 197, 204, 214, 217, 220, 223, 239, 246

aspects, 10, 12, 20, 23, 26, 30, 31, 33, 34, 40, 48, 53, 60, 62, 75, 77, 79, 86, 88, 90, 95, 97, 106, 107, 108, 109, 133, 140, 144, 151, 158, 177, 194, 221, 223, 252

Assessment, 13, 18, 21, 24, 26, 34, 51, 54, 66, 68, 70

Baseline, 148, 150

BMI, 42, 45, 46, 49, 112, 144, 145, 146, 148, 167, 171, 176, 182, 183, 188

Capabilities, 12, 15, 20, 23, 145, 149, 150

Carbohydrates, 115

Change, 4, 6, 199, 210, 212

Cholesterol, 122, 157

Circumstances, 100

Cognitive Capacities, 204

Commitment, 6, 7, 80, 103, 253

Complex Carbs, 116, 117

Conditions, 93, 104, 106, 145, 252

Consequences, 53

Conviction, 26, 30, 74, 79

Coordination, 149, 150

Develop Your Strategy, 86, 165, 171

Devise Your Plans, 87

Driving forces, 8

Eating Patterns, 151

Emotional Energy, 9

Endurance, 149

Energy Balance, 111, 133, 145, 150, 169

Essential Nutrients, 115

Establish Your Baseline, 86, 144, 145

Excuses, 216

Factors, 41

Fats, 115, 121, 128, 141

Fiber, 115, 126

Fitness, 1, 2, 1, 3, 5, 6, 7, 15, 47, 61, 65, 66, 70, 80, 88, 93, 107, 140, 145, 148, 149, 150, 157, 167, 171, 172, 198, 199, 219, 245, 246, 247

Flexibility, 140, 149, 204, 209, 260

Food, 2, 15, 49, 95, 100, 128, 133, 178, 184, 186, 198, 219, 243

Forging, 200, 201, 202

Habits, 5, 98, 101, 102, 143, 203, 210, 212, 253

Habitual Thinking, 97

Health Condition, 94

Impact, 54, 68, 108

Key Nutrients, 128

Lessons Learned, 249

Lifestyle, 145, 155, 175, 177, 230

Locations, 96

Maintenance, 5, 6, 245, 247, 248

Mastering, 222, 224

Meaning, 91

Medications, 99

Minerals, 115, 125

Momentum, 216, 217

Monounsaturated Fat, 122

Mood, 97, 100

Needs, 70, 98

Observing, 217, 218

Occasions, 95

People, 12, 50, 65, 85, 95, 96, 108, 138, 151, 178, 213

Physical Activity, 137, 138, 175, 176, 188, 189, 190, 231, 234, 243

Plans, 175

Polyunsaturated Fat, 121

Possibilities, 60

Preparation, 5, 6, 85, 86

Protein, 115, 119

Protocols, 1, 2, 1, 5, 6, 7, 80, 246

Pushback, 8

Pushbacks, 7, 252

Readiness, 10, 26, 27

RHR, 145, 146, 167

Risks, 37, 39, 47

RMR, 145, 146, 148

Saturated Fat, 121

Schedule, 186, 189, 190, 227, 243

Setup and Integration, 193, 194, 196

Simple Carbs, 115, 118

Strength, 143, 149

Takeaways, 141

Targets, 165, 167, 169

Techniques, 252

the Basics, 86, 88, 103, 165

The Situation, 95

Tools, 218, 252

Tricks, 252

Tweaking, 222, 243

Vitamins, 115, 124, 142

Water, 115, 127, 130, 143, 263

# About the Author

According to statistics kept by the National Weight Control Registry, Epi Torres is one of very few individuals who have been able to accomplish lasting weight loss and fitness improvement.

Epi was born and raised in Ponce, Puerto Rico. He holds a 1979 Bachelor's Degree in Electronics Engineering Technology from the Capitol Institute of Technology in Maryland. In 2005, the International Society of Neuro-Semantics (ISNS) certified him as an Associate Certified Meta-Coach (ACMC).

After college, he joined his father's electronic retail business (Epitronics) in Puerto Rico as a Store Manager.

In 1981, Epi left the family business to join Westinghouse Electric as an Engineer where he ascended through the management ranks and spent fifteen very successful years.

In 1997, he became Chief Operating Officer of Pittsburgh-based Contemporary Technologies, Inc.

In 2005, Epi became CEO of CTI's remote database administration services division, Remote DBA Experts.

In 2010, he took time off from running his business in order to finish this book, which he started writing in 2003. In addition, he is also developing several fitness and business Apps for the iPad platform.

He has lived in Pittsburgh, PA since 1987.

www.ingramcontent.com/pod-product-compliance
Lightning Source LLC
Chambersburg PA
CBHW060837280326
41934CB00007B/816